"*A Mother of Thousan*

shadows and plant roots of hope in your heart that will give new life to your soul."

If you have ever searched for someone who understands the loss and ache of longing for, waiting for, praying for, and not having a child, then every page in *A Mother of Thousands* was written just for you!

With vulnerability and compassion, Heather Yates shares her journey of infertility, along with her doubts, questions, grief, and the strains and struggles it brought to her marriage and her faith. Woven together with stories from Scripture and other women's journeys, Heather offers hope, courage, and a friend to lean on as she shares how the pain that almost crushed her ended up creating in her a new dream—with new hope and a new vision of motherhood more beautiful than she ever imagined!

—**Renee Swope**, award-winning author of *A Confident Heart* and former Proverbs 31 Ministries Executive Director and Radio Show Co-Host

Heather DeJesus Yates writes an honest but encouraging account of the struggle with barrenness. In this, she joins many women of the Bible who have wrestled with the same pain. Whether you are married or single, this book is a helpful book to read if your hopes for motherhood have not bloomed the way you had anticipated. You will find much solace in these pages.

—**Carolyn McCulley**, author of *Radical Womanhood* and *The Measure of Success*

As a woman who wrestled with infertility for many years, this is the book that I wish I could have read at that horrific time in my life. Heather's heart for women who are struggling with barrenness is profoundly wise, richly compassionate, and lovingly understanding. Heather's own experience with infertility will encourage brokenhearted women to believe again, to hope again, and to know that our good, good Father is at work behind the scenes in the middle of devastating disappointment.

However, let's take this one step deeper than the inability to conceive and to carry new life within one's womb. Are you disappointed that your life is not more fertile? Are you discouraged because the fruit of your labor seems dry and wasted? Heather will speak to that kind of pain as well. *A Mother of Thousands* is not just for women dealing with infertility, but it is for all of us who are ravenous for joy and hope amid the wilderness days of life.

This is a book that you will read again and again—and that you will give to others who are dealing with their own despair.

—**Carol McLeod**, author of *Stormproof* and many others

To those who have ever walked through the pain of infertility, this book will encourage your heart. But this narrative is more than just about the struggle of a barren womb. Whether you have been blessed with biological or adoptive children, this story speaks to all the shadows in our lives that loom over us as women to steal our joy.

If you feel you are living without purpose, *A Mother of Thousands* will call you out of the shadows and plant roots of hope in your heart that will give new life to your soul. *A Mother of Thousands* speaks to the revolutionary mother in all of us—barren or fertile. Read it and find new hope!

—**Julie Wilkerson Klose**, author, *Giving Hope an Address*

When we traverse the terrain of uncertainty, we often experience painful seasons that pull on our hope. Is it possible to trust God when we're staring down closed doors and are stretched to our limits? As Heather shares her story of infertility and God's provision, we see His faithfulness in ours. Perspective from Scripture and other brave mamas provide a road map for the journey. Drink deeply—your soul will thank you.

—**Angela Donadio**, author of
Finding Joy When Life is Out of Focus

A Mother of Thousands is a heartfelt extension of what Heather has long urged of me personally: to see myself as a mother in the faith even though I don't have children. The term "mother," even in the spiritual sense, was a painful reminder of all that I will never be. But Heather breaks down the walls around the different types of mothering, and brings fresh hope to women seeking to matter to someone, somewhere. She speaks knowingly from the hard places, with an honest look at who we really are in Christ.

—**Lois Martin**, Global Outreach Director,
Grace Fellowship Church

A Mother of Thousands: From Barren to Revolutionary

Published by:
Bridge-Logos
Newberry, Florida 32669, USA
www.bridgelogos.com

Printed in the United States of America

ISBN: 978-1-61036-405-8

Library of Congress Control Number: 2019932104

Edited by Lynn Copeland

Cover by Kent Jensen | knail.com

Cover photo by Tracey Hocking on Unsplash.com

Bio photo by Tara Hodges Photography

Interior design and layout by Genesis Group

All emphasis within Scripture has been added by the author.

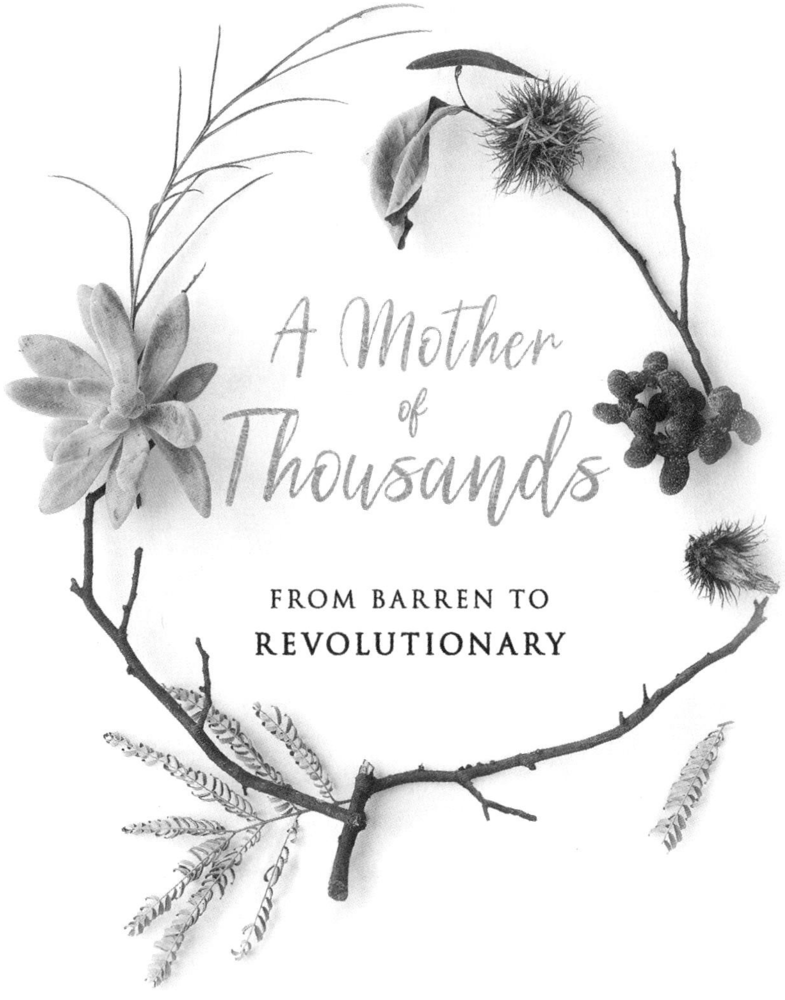

A Mother of Thousands

FROM BARREN TO REVOLUTIONARY

HEATHER DEJESUS YATES

BRIDGE LOGOS

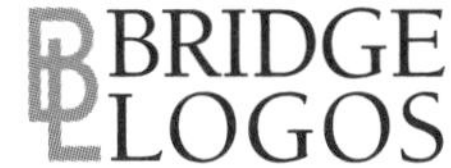

Newberry, FL 32669

For all the mamas
who do not see it yet

Contents

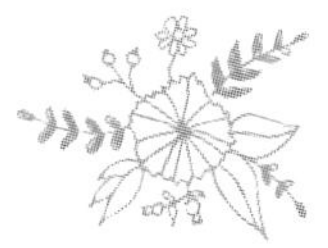

INTRODUCTION

A Mother of Thousands

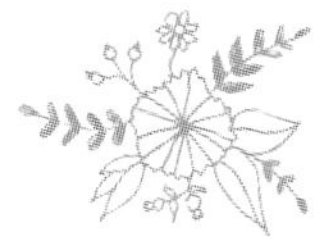

According to plant folks, there is an attractive houseplant in the succulent family that grows tiny baby plantlets (just stop and enjoy that word a bit: *plantlets*) called *a mother of thousands.*

These baby plantlets grow all along the edges of the leaves, at every tip where she branches out, until eventually they grow too heavy and drop, producing a new plant of the same kind. It is often recommended to contain these plants because of their highly "invasive" reproductive ways—and if you grow *a mother of thousands* outdoors, be forewarned that she will take over the yard. A local nursery expert cautioned planting *a mother of thousands* because one would need "good luck stopping her." Did you hear that?

She can bring about revolution.

Where once a yard may have been barren of plant life, a *mother of thousands* can bring about dramatic change that spreads without end! But here is the kicker: *a mother of thousands* plant cannot produce seed. Did you hear that too?

She is barren.

The creative God of all things plant and person can bring about a mighty unstoppable change to our communities—a *revolution*—even from the barren. Where we see an inability to bring life, whether due to a broken womb or a broken soul, God sees the potential for generations in our forever family.

Where a curse on God's creation means we endure endless weeds and empty wombs, we have a real hope in Jesus who is at work reversing the curse by redeeming our stories for God's glory and our joy.

When my husband, Jonathan, and I learned we were part of the "unexplained infertility" community, I discovered a hornet's nest of beliefs that pierced me with their stings of hopelessness.

"Heather, *you* cannot create life . . ."

"Heather, you are a *failure* as a wife . . ."

"Heather, you will *miss* your best life . . ."

My journey into infertility grief triggered the release of other wells of doubt and sadness I had not fully poured out before God. I entered a crisis of faith as my emotions swelled in that season, some days unhinging me from what I once believed was true without question. I began to sink into a secret misery over the loss of my dream of motherhood, and let shame wash over me for being unworthy of God's favor in bearing children. At the time, there were no books I could find to help me get my bearings with this kind of grief. Some books offered statistics, or explained how to get pregnant, or led me back to spiritual disciplines, but nothing climbed inside me and sat with me in the middle of infertility heartache. This was not the worst thing, as it drove me to take my grief to God in the pages of His Book, where I found hope in the written stories of Hannah, Sarah, and Anna the widow. But I wanted to hear more stories of women finding their way back to hope in this situation.

I asked God for women to meet with in person, and thankfully found these women existed right in my own community! Soon, a holy gathering of half a dozen women with infertility stories began to form around a dinner table, nearly monthly. We shared stories of where we grew up, and how. We eagerly leaned toward each other for the details of how we met our husbands, savoring all the tasty bits. We slowly and somberly waded through the diagnoses, the miscarriages, the infertility treatments, the tears shed, the conversations had, the whispered prayers, the adoption paperwork, the pounding of hearts in hospital rooms waiting to hear birthparents' decisions. We talked about language, how adoption feels, how seeing baby bumps triggers sadness, how we view God with us in all of it. In that little community I found what I wanted in a book. I found the voices of women who could say without fear of being misunderstood: I hate it. I hate it. I hate it. Then with the next breath say, without fear of being dismissed: But I have hope here too.

So precious reader, this is *that* book. This is a book for women who feel barren, who believe they are unable to create meaningful lives due to either a broken womb or a broken soul. This is a book that says of barrenness: I hate it, I hate it, I hate it. And in the next breath says: But I have hope here too.

WHO YOU ARE

I'm going to assume we all want to live meaningful lives, right? We want a life filled with meaning, in contrast to a wasted life with no lasting meaning. When I believed I couldn't create life, I felt like much of what I did was a waste. If what I did wasn't building toward my dream of being a mother of children, what did it matter? What did any of my other efforts in life matter? And let me stretch a little further and confess this rock-bottom zinger: If I couldn't bear children I felt (even for just a little while) like *I* was a waste.

Thankfully, if there's one thing we can count on with Jesus (there are countless things we can count on Him for, by the way), it is that He wastes nothing! Jesus can take every pain and produce meaning, including infertility grief. Jesus doesn't invite us into a competitive race of living *the most* meaningful life, as if there was one kind of meaning, with limited space for runners. Getting married and having babies that look like us is not the only kind of meaningful life out there. Instead, Jesus calls us to a completely different way of looking at life fundamentally:

Jesus invites us to live lives of meaning by making our lives about *Him*, not us.

As people who walk the earth with Jesus as our Teacher, we carry the unstoppable seed of the gospel within our very souls. When we choose to plant the seed of Jesus' love in hearts growing near ours, we regenerate the soil of our culture. New life is born out of an old Love that loved us first. Quite literally, we can change our world by simply showing up to it, with God's transformative love. And nothing in life carries more meaning! I have discovered these hopeful truths in my journey through infertility grief:

All women can live uniquely meaningful lives.

Christ in us makes us capable of bearing life spiritually —so we can *all* become mothers!

We can be revolutionaries—we can join God in changing our world.

Yet change sometimes seems impossible, and no matter how hard we try, we can still *feel* stuck and hopeless. Ultimately, as long as we are on this side of eternity, we will still feel the weight of the curse on this earth, on our bodies, on our relationships. So I wrestled with this truth in my journey through infertility grief, too:

Not all women can live the *same* meaningful life.

A curse on earth brings obstacles to bearing life.

We are all spiritually barren apart from Jesus.

Out of the depths of my own infertility grief, my heartaches and joys with adoption and fostering, and a desperate pursuit of hope of living *my* meaningful life, God gave me a new vision for motherhood—one where every woman can find her place as a *mother*. But it won't come about automatically; we will need to *choose* to move through our grief and embrace this vision with our whole heart. We will become women with grit—for a heated battle ensues to contain us!

So who are you, dear reader? You may be a woman who has received all the negative pregnancy tests, has lost babies through miscarriage or death, has experienced failed adoptions—or has believed childless is *less*. You are a woman tempted to doubt you can leave a rich and meaningful legacy now. Or you are a woman with children, but you still feel empty, dry, barren in your soul, wondering why you aren't a more "*joyful* mother of children" (Psalm 113:9). Or you may be a woman wanting to come alongside one of these women, and to you I say *thank you* for your gentle compassion. But you also may be a man, wondering how to move forward with your own questions to help a woman in your life who needs your strength. Know I am praying for all of you, wherever you are at today, that you find hope in these pages and on your journey.

WHAT TO EXPECT IN THESE PAGES

My faith in God, His Son Jesus, and His Holy Spirit within me were my immovable anchors throughout my journey with infertility grief and continue to hold me to the shore of hope. I could not, nor did I have any inclination to, write this book with any other mooring. I hope that as you read you are able to hear the heart of a woman who wants to find a place for sorrow and peace and finds it with the help of God and others. I assume you are reading this book because you are looking for hope yourself, and are curious to hear what Scripture and other women's stories offer us. With that said, I have structured this book around three main elements:

our *humanity* | our *spirituality* | our *destiny*

Every person with breath shares these three elements. We are all human. We feel pain and grieve and delight and dance. We are at the same time spiritual. Created in the image of God, we are born with a body, soul, and spirit (1 Thessalonians 5:23). Due to the curse of sin on the earth brought on by Adam and Eve's disobedience in the beginning of our shared human history, our spiritual nature is separated from God, dead and in need of resurrection to new life. God made a way for our spiritual resurrection by sending His only Son, Jesus Christ, to live a sinless life, die on a cross for our sins, and be buried in a tomb for three days before rising from the dead (1 Corinthians 15:1–5). Now, any person who puts their trust in Jesus Christ as Savior and Lord experiences a spiritual rebirth by faith. The spirit that was once dead in sin becomes alive with Christ, who comes to dwell in each of us (Romans 8:10,11). And third, every person has a destiny, a forever ahead as a spiritual being. In the image of God we are created as eternal beings, and for those born again in Christ, this eternity with Him is now secured by Him.

I wanted to share my journey with infertility grief by coming up out of the pages of my human pain to see it the way God sees it: in the fuller light of my humanity, my spirituality, and my destiny. This perspective helped me, and I am hoping it helps you see your story in a fresh way too. I also refer to different seasons of my life throughout the chapters, so to give you a clearer context for the stories you will read, here is a brief chronology of the seasons of my life to serve you along the way:

- After law school I worked in a law firm where we practiced adoption law, among other things, and I dreamed of adopting someday. I left the practice after several years to work at the Florida Legislature, and also began serving pregnant teens and women at risk of homelessness in that community.
- In 2008, Jonathan and I married and I moved to Tennessee, where I practiced law briefly before transitioning into vocational women's ministry at our church. There we became diagnosed with unexplained infertility and began infertility treatments.
- After several failed attempts to conceive with treatments, we chose to pursue adoption through an agency. We started a journey to adopt two children, one domestically and one internationally. I also started a blog to chronicle our journey and share what I was learning with God.
- In 2014 we brought home a beautiful daughter born domestically! Many wonderful and challenging things took place in our adoption story, and impacted our international adoption journey.
- To heal from infertility grief and post-adoptive trauma, I left my job and withdrew from my blog and almost all social media.

- We fostered for a time, and experienced a failed adoption of twin boys before finally embracing our family complete as a threesome.

As I tell my story, you will find references to Scriptures, as well as casual language I use in describing my relationship with God. With the depth of emotions I had to wade through at times, I needed to tell this story simply in my own way. You'll find stories of other women told in Scripture too, as well as themes like discipleship. If this isn't interesting to you, I urge you to see it through to the end because you may be surprised by how our human and spiritual natures work together in some amazing ways!

While you could read through this book quickly and pull from it encouragement, connection, and even healing, I want this book to be a transformational tool for you. When it comes to our beliefs, before we can plant new seeds full of truth, sometimes we need to first uproot beliefs that are no longer helpful, that are hindering growth or are outright false. So at the end of each chapter, I give you ideas for what may need to be uprooted in your mind and what is worth planting before moving forward. If you choose to use these ideas, take these steps prayerfully, knowing that all seed takes time to appear. Don't be fooled into disbelief when you don't see change in your mind or heart overnight! This isn't the way in nature, and it is not the way in people either. Simply keep uprooting lies, and keep planting truth, and you *will* be taking next steps in becoming *a mother of thousands*. God promises that in due time a good harvest *will* come in for your soul when you root yourself in God's love:

> "If you abide in Me, and My words abide in you, you will ask what you desire, and it shall be done for you. By this My Father is glorified, that you bear *much fruit;* so you will be My

> disciples. As the Father loved Me, I also have loved you; abide in My love." (John 15:7–9)

In this book you will not only find my infertility story and the stories of famous "barren women" in Scripture, you will hear from other women with infertility stories too. Nearly a dozen women offered to share with you their grief and God's glory in their journey. This may be my deepest joy in this project: seeing women raise their voices not to brag on their own courage—though they are courageous—but to hopefully connect with your pain and point to God for their hope. These women have endured loss, held secret miseries, have made choices to love, and have drawn others closer to Jesus because of the grace in their testimonies. I consider it a high privilege to share space on the page with these women, and I hope by hearing other voices, you can find your own. More than anything, though, I hope you hear God's voice speaking words of life and hope for *you*.

LAST CALL

This world won't stay open all night, friends. I don't mean to be dramatic (it just comes naturally), but this could be our last call. The enemy of God and of our souls would love nothing more than for us to stay consumed in pain and grief over our infertility, or stuck in feelings of barrenness. Women, I believe now is the time for us to bravely show up to our generation with our gifts and our grief, our passion and our pain, our creativity and our curiosity, our on-trend and our ordinary because with Jesus living *in* us, there is no stopping *His* reproductive ways through us!

We are the daughters of Eve—redeemed. The curse happened, yes, but so did a cross. Now motherhood is for *all* of us. Women, we are made to bear life!

May this book comfort those of you struggling with infertility, but also call you out of the shadows of shame and grief as we choose together to take our place in this call of motherhood, in our generation.

For those feeling spiritually barren, may this book shake you awake to the distractions of comparison, the lies of worthlessness, and the temptation for retirement, and keep you from facing a finish line with regret. May your souls find here nourishing truth reminding you that *you* have vibrant life-bearing power yet within you!

May we all look up to the bigger story God is scripting out in our lives. May we all engage the battle against us in barrenness, in body, soul, and spirit, and fight with our faith in the God who created us to be fruitful, multiply, and fill the earth! May each of us experience the eternal joy of getting to say:

I am *a mother of thousands.*

PART ONE

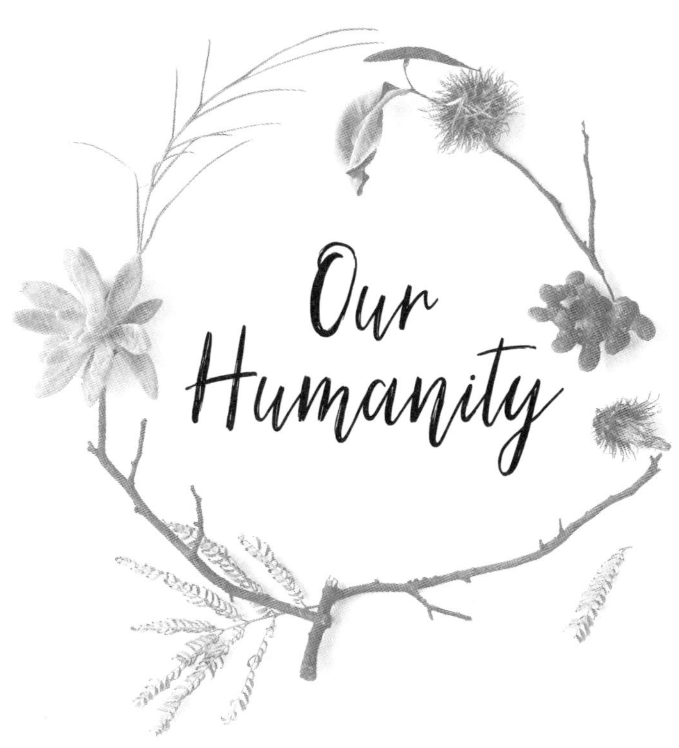

Our Humanity

CHAPTER 1

The Membership No Woman Seeks

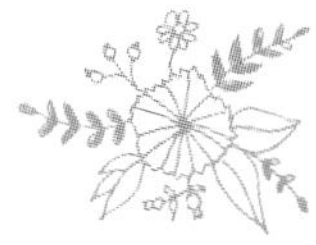

Peninnah had children, but Hannah had no children.

—1 SAMUEL 1:2

Infertility is one of those topics no woman wants to be qualified to write on in first-person. No one wants to suffer the loss of a dream. And yet, we are grateful for the brave ones who put pain to paper, who share the story behind their personal struggle. We turn the pages listening not so much for the author's voice, but for signs of ours echoing back to us. We long to feel understood and not alone. Often it is when we are looking into others' stories that we discover light filling our own.

While I have hope that telling of our struggle here will help you, this wasn't the book I pitched to my publisher. The book I was prepared to write was a devotional. It had been on my mind for years, and I thought this was the time to go for it. But for over a week the contract remained untouched on my desk. I couldn't figure out why I was hesitant. Then a podcast aired of an interview I had done months earlier with the launch of my first book. I talked about our journey with infertility and adoption. People started listening to it and sharing it. It was resonating deeply with women, so I decided to blog on the topic and highlight the show.

Then *more* responses came in, now to the blog post as well.

- "Heather, women need to hear this who are struggling with infertility pain. Your story could offer a lot of people comfort, and hope."
- "I'm crying reading your blog post."
- "I just finished the podcast, I needed that so much, you don't even know."

When you begin to notice a current of voices saying the same thing, from every direction, sometimes wisdom says fold up the blueprint and go back to the drawing board with God. He may have new plans!

Friends, this is what you hold in your hands: God's new plan for my second book.

And really, what a fitting introduction to this book. This is an infertility story that started with a barren woman who, thanks to God's new plan, became a revolutionary.

WHAT DO I MEAN BY "REVOLUTIONARY"?

A revolutionary is one who is "bringing about a major or fundamental change."[1] Another definition includes "involving or causing a complete or dramatic change" in a status quo.[2] The status quo in this case is a vision of motherhood that consists only of women who parent children in their home—either birthed from their bellies or not, but especially those who get pregnant and deliver children.

This book puts this status quo in a deep stretch and makes the case that motherhood is for *all* women—even the barren.

One reason I didn't plan to write this book is that discussing my infertility wasn't even on my radar. I share about infertility on my blog in patches, and I mentioned it some in my first book, *All the Wild Pearls*. But until now I haven't made it a feature conversation because, well, my life is about so much more than that one thing.

We are more than our losses!

There was a time, though, when I didn't feel this way. There was a season when infertility was the headline of every story in my mind. In fact, for years infertility pain made it hard to tune in to anything else. I wouldn't have written this book back then because I couldn't have—I was feeling my way through the dark of it with God. Or, I was denying it was even true for us. In short: *this wasn't the book I wanted to write because the life I imagined with infertility was not the life I wanted to live.* The infertility club was not the membership I wanted to join. I had to grieve my way through the pain of the loss, and had no way of knowing where I'd end up or what I'd face on the other side—*if* there was another side.

The infertility club was not the membership I wanted to join.

And while this book doesn't end with one of those surprise "rainbow baby" pregnancies like many infertility resources offer, I can share a journey that somehow, mysteriously, and imperfectly but triumphantly has brought me out into the light again!

Pastor Timothy Keller once said, "If we knew what God knows, we would ask exactly for what he gives."[3] Another way of saying (or seeing) this is in terms of God's will, which has been a difficult concept for me to peacefully understand: *God's will is what we would want if we could see what God sees.*

With this I can agree. When my lens makes God appear as He is—mighty *and* good—the whole of Scripture, and especially suffering, makes a little more sense to me. And in my own way this is what I hope to do for you: give you a new lens through which you see God, yourself, your story, and this membership.

STILL NOT CONVINCED

I wish I could say I faithfully set sail on writing this book after choosing to follow God's new plan. But even after getting the contract with this new book title, I still hesitated. I wasn't sure I had the emotional energy to feel these chapters of my story, let alone write about them further. After much prayer and discussion with my husband and a few others, I decided to sign the contract and send it in even with my hesitations. That was a Wednesday night, September 13, 2018.

Within two weeks I started second-guessing my decision to write this book, again, wondering if I had rushed ahead of God. I feared I was now headlong onto a path that was not only going to feel miserable, it was going to produce weeds and thistles in the hearts of others. I wrestled with a pit in my stomach for a couple of days before I bowed my knees in prayer. With my mind racing down two lanes at once, and my heart bulging with anxiety, I bent down and prayerfully cried out my surrender. I surrendered to whatever it was God wanted with me, just as long as He would speak to me. After several quiet minutes I got up off the floor faintly trusting He could answer my prayer.

The next morning I sat to read my Bible and continued to pray for direction. I sensed a nudge to read Psalm 114. After reading through it once, I went back to the beginning to read it again out loud. This time, I noticed the verse above it, in Psalm 113. It was a lone verse circled, starred, and dated. I read the verse and immediately my soul flipped inside of itself—I knew the God of the universe was knocking on my door. This was what I read:

> He grants *the barren* woman a home, like a joyful mother of children. (Psalm 113:9)

Can you believe it? A verse about infertility! I felt God confirmed that it was time to talk about this journey, and even to use the word "barren" in the book title, a word I resisted because of the shame it can carry. But that is not all. After I read the verse, I looked to the side and saw the date written when that verse had first meant something to me: September 13, 2016.

God had prepared *this* book, two years prior to the date on my contract.

Friend, I don't know why you are picking up this book to read. I don't know if you have an infertility story, or someone you love is struggling with grief. But I have no doubt anymore that God has a plan for *this* message—and for you!

LET'S SKIP THE SCIENCE LESSON

If you are looking for a book on the science and statistics of infertility, this is not that book, mainly because numbers mean very little to a heart that is hurting. You also won't find tips for how to reverse infertility because, though I applied many of them, I'm clearly no expert. This book then will skip the science and focus more on your soul. What you will find is how I have worked through infertility heartache, and even still continue to bring it to God. I aimed to share as openly as I could, for your sake, without dishonoring my family. If it is something *good* to share for building you up, making connection with you and offering comfort, you will find it in these pages. I'm not a licensed counselor, though. This book is not meant to substitute for the soul care you may need this season with a professional therapist, but I hope it will support your journey.

In this book I will give you nothing that I haven't first received myself from God. I'm not just some loving woman who wants to be good to people, though this is who I want to become. In the pit of barrenness I hated everyone. I was angry and felt bitter toward women who conceived effortlessly. I believed many things about God that were not true because of what felt like rejection of me and favoritism for others. One of many truths I learned from God, that has brought me comfort with infertility, is found in the book of Samuel. It is a story of two women: Peninnah, who was able to conceive children, and Hannah, who was loved by her husband though "the LORD had closed her womb" (1 Samuel 1:5). A rivalry ensued between the women as Peninnah (the childbearing wife of Elkanah) "provoked her [Hannah] severely, to make her miserable, because the LORD had closed her womb." Scripture records that "year by year" when Hannah went to the house of the LORD, she was continually provoked by Peninnah so that she was moved to weeping, unable to eat (1 Samuel 1:7). Hannah is described as being in "bitterness of soul" as she prayed to the LORD and "wept in anguish" (1 Samuel 1:10).

We all wrestle with misunderstandings of the love of God and with broken dreams.

When you are walking through an infertility story, you may feel like a Hannah in a world of Peninnahs, even those who do not mean to cause pain. Social media inflames sorrow with images of baby bumps, baby announcements, and welcome-to-the-world celebrations. It is natural for a woman to rejoice in her blessings; we all have blessings that others may desire, yet lack. It's not that you don't wish pregnancies on friends; it's just that the pain can feel so intense with longing and grief that it is bittersweet to witness that particular celebration. We want to be women who celebrate with each other, but we need to find a path for living in the tension of celebration and longing.

One way I found hope in this tension was to follow Hannah's pattern. I followed her steps and continually went to God with weeping and occasionally fasting in prayer. In her shoes, I noticed how Peninnah had anguish and insecurity, too. She felt unloved by her husband, and seeing Hannah's blessing pierced her with grief of her own. Both women had reason to celebrate. Both women had reason to grieve. In their own ways, both women felt unable to create life. So here is the rub: we all feel insecure and rejected on some level. We all wrestle with misunderstandings of the love of God and with broken dreams. We all provoke one another, whether we mean to or not.

In the height of my "bitterness of soul" I was unable to see the longing and grief in other women's lives. My loss felt like cruelty, as if God were choosing to bless other women because He loved them more. I felt the closed womb of Hannah, but I also felt the rejection of Peninnah. But the truth was God never took His love or His purposes away from me by inviting me into this membership. And He hasn't taken them away from you either.

What I can offer you in the chapters that follow is the comfort I received from this God who loves and purposes, who closes and opens doors, and who always wants the best for us. I pray God multiplies this hope I found in the hearts of everyone who reads this book, too.

Blessed be the God and Father of our Lord Jesus Christ, the Father of mercies and God of all comfort, who comforts us in all our tribulation, that we may be able to comfort those who are in any trouble, with the comfort with which we ourselves are comforted by God. For as the sufferings of Christ abound in us, so our consolation also abounds through Christ. (2 Corinthians 1:3–5)

Joanna's Story

When I was a little girl and people asked me what I wanted to be when I grew up, I replied, "A mommy." I never really imagined what kind of job I would do for a living, much less a career, so I was shocked at the start of my junior year when my university advisor strongly suggested I choose a major. I married the man of my dreams two weeks after graduation, and just planned on working for a few years until we had our first child. We both wanted me to be a stay-at-home mom, and I was thrilled at the possibilities of library story time, "mommy and me" music and yoga, infant massage classes, and play groups.

I'd heard stories of friends struggling to get pregnant but had no advice to offer, and honestly skipped women's magazine articles on infertility or miscarriage because this would never be *my* story. I had a plan! Be a stay-at-home mom, with a smoking hot husband, a sweet little dog, 2.5 kids, and a white picket fence. We were completely caught off guard when my doctor referred us to a fertility specialist. I couldn't even think about the word "infertility" without crying. I just kept thinking that surely there was a mistake. This couldn't be happening to me. This wasn't how my story was supposed to go.

We decided to share our struggles with our parents and a few close friends. We experienced two very close deaths in our immediate families, and because of this so much of our early married life was public knowledge. I didn't want others to know and perhaps I was in a state of shock. I thought maybe the first referral appointment would be our "test of faith" and we would find that I was, in fact, pregnant. I had heard other stories of this, so it can happen, right? But after tests confirmed I was indeed not pregnant, the fertility specialist suggested we move forward with some mildly aggressive treatments. I was devastated. I felt like we had done something "wrong" and were being punished and didn't know why. My darkness and despair over childlessness and this new struggle to conceive created a breeding ground for arguments, tears, and bitterness within our marriage.

My husband is a fixer, and infertility was something completely out of his hands to fix. I felt so isolated and alone. Everyone around me was either pregnant or had a newborn, and I was green with envy. I searched all the websites, clinging to new procedures with high success rates, or to stories of women who faced infertility but ultimately conceived. The inner critic was so harsh. Was I being punished? Did God not love me? Did we make a mistake in marrying each other? Was my faith not strong enough? I cried and begged for God to help me to get pregnant. I told Him I would share our story with anyone who asked or struggled if He would only give us a pregnancy with a healthy baby at the end. I didn't need 2.5 children—one is perfect, God. Just give me one.

After the mildly and then moderately aggressive treatments ended in miscarriage and loss, we felt broken—emotionally, spiritually, and financially. I was so angry with God. Why would He put us through all this? I stopped talking to Him and, much like Jonah, I tried to hide from Him. My husband and I grieved separately and yet also together. I truly felt like this was the end of my story. Something must be wrong with me. I cannot carry or deliver/create a life, so what good am I to anyone? God didn't love me, and He had ignored my dreams of becoming a mother.

I decided to shift my thoughts and focused on graduate school and my career. I slowly began to feel God's presence in my life again. I felt nudges to encourage a friend, look at a situation through a different lens, and find joy in every day. I realized my hope was never to be built on a baby. My hope is in Christ. I began to realize that I was never alone in my suffering. He is Immanuel. He is God *with* us. He was there all along. He was at every appointment, held my hand through every shot and procedure, and was with us when we received devastating news. He wiped every tear, and continues to. He had a purpose in our journey. He is faithful and wants good things for His children. We just have to take the next step and trust that He is with us, and that He is faithful always.

UPROOT

What do you tend to believe about God, yourself, and your circumstances, when what *you* planned doesn't go as planned?

PLANT

Consider this statement: "God's will is what you would want if you could see what God sees." How could believing this enable you to see your "changed" plans differently?

CHAPTER 2

Denial, Doctors, and Donuts

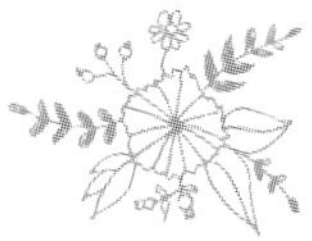

So Hannah ate.

—1 SAMUEL 1:9 (MSG)

Ironically, I have avoided writing this chapter because I have simply not wanted to deal with the emotions and confessions that come with it. Essentially, I have been in denial about my denial. Real mature, right? We deny things for a reason, though. In fact, it's very sensible to avoid our wounds. Pain hurts, so nothing in our being wants to move toward pain willingly. When my daughter skins her knee, she brushes away all efforts to bring aid and healing. Contact is unthinkable because the wound hurts. She doesn't understand that moving toward the wound with the right treatment in love will bring recovery. She doesn't care about recovery; she cares about not feeling any additional pain in that moment. Don't we all relate on some level? When we are in crisis, pain becomes an enemy to avoid, not a helpful cue that care is needed for wholeness. All my daughter wants to do in those moments is brace herself. I think she believes she can somehow absorb the pain, ignore the wound, and move on with her life.

In my own way, this is what I did for years with my infertility grief.

THE DIAGNOSIS

My husband, Jonathan, and I met through the online dating service eHarmony. I was thirty when we met and thirty-one when we married. We dated only a few months before we were engaged, and then were engaged only seven months before we were married. Our courtship was one of the sweetest seasons of our lives, watching God guide us with such care. He fulfilled promises to our hearts in ways we never could have imagined. Our courtship was guided by family, friends, and mentors who prayed for us and gave wise counsel. Our union felt like a celebration of God's faithfulness! At the time, I had no doubt God would also bless our marriage with babies someday, because clearly He had gone to great lengths to bring us together! We had honored Him in our single years, waited on His provision for one another, and "did it right"... so surely God was pleased with us. Surely, children were a reward and we could expect them in due time, just as Scripture seems to promise:

> Behold, children are a heritage from the LORD, the fruit of the womb is a reward. Like arrows in the hand of a warrior, so are the children of one's youth. Happy is the man who has his quiver full of them; they shall not be ashamed, but shall speak with their enemies in the gate. (Psalm 127:3–5)

Since we had been together for less than a year when we married, we wanted to invest in our relationship for a couple of years before extending ourselves as parents. I felt a little nervous about waiting too long to try to have children, since I was already in my early thirties, but we had agreed at the start that our marriage was our priority and that we would serve children better by building a strong foundation for ourselves. (This has since proved to still be one of our wisest choices, as our marriage has had to bear some heavy burdens in its ten-year lifespan!) Then at age thirty-three, we received the all-clear from our doctors that we were in great shape to start trying to build a family, and we were both expectant that we would be expecting any day!

> Then God blessed them, and God said to them, "Be fruitful and multiply; fill the earth and subdue it..." (Genesis 1:28)

Right out of the gate, in that first month, I actually showed some signs of being pregnant. I was ecstatic. A dear family friend was on the same timeline as we were, seeking to get pregnant. We were sharing prayers and she was sensing she might be pregnant that first month too! It was around Christmas time and I thought, "This would be just like God to gift us with this great news at Christmas!" But a week later we realized it was either a loss of a child or a loss of a hope, for us. My friend consequently received the joyful news that she was indeed pregnant.

Though I was obviously sad and disappointed, I thought the second month would be different. But the second month came and went with nothing. Then the third, the fourth, the fifth...and with every month that passed my emotions grew more intense. I would both swell higher with hope that *this* would be the month and then would fall deeper into sadness when I discovered it was *not* the month. I started buying books, reading blogs, and asking friends for whatever tips I could find on *how to conceive*. I wasn't so obsessed with getting pregnant that I talked of nothing else, but it certainly occupied the majority of my mental and emotional space.

During that first year of trying to conceive I was leading Bible studies for women and speaking at events at my church. I had desires to write and speak on issues that mattered to me, and even taught women how to advocate for women and family issues before our US Congress. I was not actively looking to build a career around these passions at that time, though, because we were hoping to build our family. I had dreamed of many things, including being a mom at home for a season, ever since I was a child. Jonathan was willing to support any of my dreams, so we chose to base our budget on his income alone so we would have flexibility. I didn't recognize this belief at the time, but since I was serving God and was not earning an income, I subtly expected to get the desires of my heart fulfilled (as I knew them): to have a baby. The problem with unaddressed expectations is that when they aren't met, hurt happens. And you'll see soon how *poorly* I handle hurt.

The only thing reproducing in me was fear and a litany of questions with no clear answers.

After the twelfth month passed with no pregnancy, it was time to return for my annual physical. I remember leaving the house, making the drive, parking the car, and weighing in. The last time I sat in my doctor's office I had all the hope in the world of being pregnant soon. I had expected to make this trip for an ultrasound on my pregnant belly. Even on this visit I held on to a thin hope that maybe she would have a quick fix or word of encouragement with some statistic I missed that gives hope for the second year of trying to conceive. Instead, her face said it all. She didn't have any answers or encouraging word for me, but only a referral to a local *infertility* specialist. The word felt like broken glass going into my ears, cutting tissue all the way to my brain.

Infertility is defined in many ways, but at the root the definition carries this concept: "the failure to achieve a clinical pregnancy within twelve months or more." Do you hear the hurtful words? *Failure to achieve.* My husband and I both rank "Achiever" on our top five strengths according to the StrengthsFinder assessment.[4] We also both identify as Type 1 on the Enneagram model, which means our basic fear is being defective or failing. The bottom line is that finding out we were a part of the "infertility" community was the toughest blow we could get for our personality types, on top of the growing grief behind our disappointment itself.

I left the appointment in a daze. I somehow made it to the car and fumbled my husband's number on my phone. I don't even remember what he said. It was probably something "glass half-full" because that is his nature, but I know a lot of tears flooded out that day on my end. Within a couple of weeks we were both sitting in the waiting room of an infertility specialist's office, with magazines of a very different nature fanned out on tiny tables next to chairs. I didn't want to read anything, though, or make eye contact with anyone, or even talk to my husband. All my energy went into holding myself together. Just beneath the surface I could feel an emotional river raging with confusion and sadness that bubbled up as anger, then sank into a soupy sorrow.

The only thing reproducing in me was fear and a litany of questions with no clear answers. As the minutes dragged in that waiting room, some of those questions would crash against my heart and ricochet in my thoughts. *How did we get here? What did I do wrong? What does this mean for our dreams of having a family? Is God testing our faithfulness? Is this God's enemy trying to hurt us? Will fertility treatments make me even crazier than I feel now? Will it hurt? What if we never conceive? Will I die alone? What would I do with my broken heart? What would I do with my time? How will I not fall apart every time I see a pregnant woman? Will Jonathan be disappointed in me? Will we make it through this together well?* I found myself unconsciously pinning each question down to a mat of denial, desperate to seem like a woman with her wits about her—at least for the next hour.

We eventually went through the basic evaluations and were cleared with having no medical reasons to explain why we were experiencing infertility. In part, we were relieved. We were labeled with "unexplained infertility." We were told statistics based on age, given pamphlets and left with options to consider for next steps along with a tiny shred of hope.

I had made it through the appointment without releasing the tidal wave of emotion this diagnosis brought with it. My willpower to stay calm was sufficient for the hour. But soon that temporarily helpful approach would turn into full-blown denial. Once again, I would acknowledge God in my hurt but would turn to an old comfort for my soul: food. And unfortunately for my waistline, a favorite donut shop was just down the road from the infertility specialist's office. Our diagnosis of "unexplained infertility" came at the best and worst season: pumpkin munchkin season! I packed up my grief and confusion in the folder with the fertility treatment options, and took my denial to Dunkin' Donuts. God would have to up His game if He was going to get anywhere close to my wound.

PAIN AND POWDERED SUGAR

Denial of hurt seems to work for a while, but as we live in these bodies we eventually learn that avoiding pain brings us no lasting comfort. Whether it's a low-grade anxiety, or a more severe emotional bondage, the source of the pain is a lie rooted in our souls. This lie pinches our emotional nerves, impacting how we think and how our body responds, and will continue pinching regardless of how much we try to numb the pain. Just as pinched nerves radiate pain to unlikely places in our bodies, unresolved grief can manifest itself in strange unhealthy behaviors that look completely unrelated. But there's more. Pain avoidance not only delays our healing, it can actually create more problems for us than we had at the start.

My classic response to uncomfortable feelings (well, comfortable ones too, let's just lay it all out there) has been to eat. Ever since I was a child, I can remember turning to food as a way of quieting the low-grade anxiety that lingered inside of me. I shared in my first book, *All the Wild Pearls*, about some childhood traumas that instilled fear in my tiny soul. When you are really young, you have no idea how to cope with pain that isn't addressed by the adults in your life. Left to your own resources, you do what you can to bring relief and stop the sensation of discomfort. So for me, relief came by way of food. First it was at my grandparents' house, but then I snuck in extra portions after dinner while cleaning the dishes. This grew to secret runs to the refrigerator or pantry when no one was watching. Later in adulthood, my coping mechanism became so deeply entrenched that food became the boss of me and feeling my pain grew more unfamiliar and dangerous.

So the cycle continued: feeling hurt, being afraid of my pain, food presenting a road of immediate comfort for fear, taking that road growing only more afraid of feeling pain, as well as ashamed for weight gain and idolatry. I would often cry out to God to help me not overeat and beg Him for help to lose weight and to walk in the self-control of His Spirit. In truth, I wanted some magical deliverance without having to deal with the root beliefs entangled with hurt in my heart. God in His mercy would soothe my distress in that moment, but later used my stubborn unrelenting infertility grief to draw me into deeper confession. I felt the tenderness of God's invitation to be healed:

> "I am the LORD your God, who brought you out . . .; open your mouth wide, and I will fill it. But My people would not heed My voice . . ." (Psalm 81:10,11)

I didn't want to listen to God's voice, especially if it meant I wasn't going to bear children. But in time, God would use the deepest sorrow of my soul to bring me into a wildly wonderful new way of living with Him, myself, and others.

THE DREADED "B" WORD

Language is mysterious. What is it about a word that gives it so much power? Some words, just the sight or sound of them, conjure up a host of stories and happy memories and inspire hope, while others ring like a death knell.

I had never really noticed the word "barren" before we faced infertility. My only experience with it was in Scripture and the association was not a good one. Barrenness in the Bible was not limited to just a personal grief for a couple; it was a dead end. Another dreaded word was associated with it: *curse*. Children were seen as a sign of material blessings, like in Psalm 127:3–5 quoted earlier. Children provided a very practical answer to the question, "Who will take care of us in old age?" Many of the leading men and women in Scripture cried out to God feeling forgotten by Him because of their infertility stories, so it leaves men and women today to wonder: *Has God forgotten me here? Can He, or does He, forget us?*

As I mentioned in chapter 1, Scripture helped me find the path of hope, not only for my infertility grief, but also for my pain avoidance. There are stories of women in Scripture who have "been there" when it comes to feeling forgotten, even cursed, by God. While we can only speculate about their family dynamics, many widely admired history-making women in Scripture are not mentioned as having children: Miriam, Esther, Priscilla, Mary and Martha, and Mary Magdalene. Whether it is because of a literal barrenness of womb, or a barrenness of soul, we can connect with these women and find a way to face our pain with Jesus. And let's be clear. You don't have to be barren of womb to feel like you have been forgotten by God or have nothing to offer. The enemy of God, and of our souls, is happy to take our experience in this fallen world, where the earth sprouts weeds and wombs sprout nothing, and make it seem like something is wrong with us. But God is always, always, *always* working in us greater freedom, and is always making *all* things new.

You don't have to be barren of womb to feel like you have been forgotten by God or have nothing to offer.

Maura's Story

My husband and I married after my twenty-fourth birthday. We had dreams that we would move from just the two of us and would start a family. I remember the first two honeymoon months we went with the flow hoping and trying to conceive. With each passing month, pressure was mounting—pressure from our own desires, from family, from cultural expectations to have babies. We were both young and healthy, so we just thought it was a matter of time. After we celebrated our first-year anniversary and engaged in the customary "how to conceive" information overload, we decided to visit a specialist.

I remember sitting in the fertility specialist's office as he read our questionnaire, having little doubt we would be one of his success stories. We shared with him that we had intercourse five or six times a week, back then. Our diets were clean, and from the outside looking in, we were healthy enough to conceive. He prescribed Clomid, with a warning that multiple births were more likely than not getting pregnant. Our pharmacist laughed a little when he gave us this and said, "Good luck."

Time passed and a couple more visits to cold, dark doctor rooms full of ultrasounds met us with, "Everything looks good," but we still couldn't conceive. I look back at that time, remembering more than ten vaginal ultrasounds in that room, as one of the cloudiest in my life, figuratively and mentally. The examining room was sterile and white with long drapes and an ultrasound machine and scope ready to probe.

After more time passed, the doctor decided to do a hysterosalpingogram (HSG) test, which he explained was a more thorough X-ray of my fallopian tubes to see why I wasn't pregnant yet. So we scheduled it. This test was done in a hospital operating room, but we were still reassured it was noninvasive. This test changed everything for our family. I remember the doctor's face clearly when he was administering the dye into my fallopian tubes. His face seemed to shrivel up, full of dread. Everyone in the room knew something was wrong and after a quick flash of a couple of pictures, the doctor turned off the dye-tracking monitor and asked that I dress. He would go over the results later.

When he walked us through the X-rays, he immediately, and without an ounce of good news, explained my tubes were blocked and not a speck of dye was able to penetrate either tube. At that moment he stamped me *infertile*. He asked that we schedule a new type of appointment at his office, an appointment to discuss in-vitro fertilization (IVF), because he believed this would be the only way for my husband and I to conceive together.

Jump ahead seven years and we were finally ready to embark on our IVF journey. Seven years of wondering why am I not "woman enough" to bear children for my husband. Seven years of wondering how ugly the inside of my body is that it doesn't want to bear life. Sadly, seven years of being upset when friends got pregnant. I would fake my excitement for each of them. I was happy for them, but jealousy became my primary emotion. With each ultrasound picture and pregnancy test, I continued in a devastated emotional coma. One joy during this time was that in these seven years, my husband reminded me of his unconditional love, that I was enough, regardless. This was a long season in the valley, but I did not know God was meeting me here.

God placed in my heart the desire to have children. He gave me a vision for how He would do this in my life, but seven long years passed before that vision would begin, and even then it was by faith, without any guarantees. To describe IVF best, I would use the term "medical pin cushion." The nurse drew two large circles on my back with a permanent marker and my husband would inject a needle into those circles, to the point he would complain that there was nowhere left in those circles without a bruise. I remember once we forgot an injection, so during my lunch break, I pulled up my shirt in our car and bent over for two more injections so as to not miss the strictly timed guidelines of each injection. And those were the ones in the back! The injections in my stomach and lower abdomen were the scariest. I remember the instructions stated the needles were just long enough to penetrate into the specific part of the muscle to not do damage to my intestines!

The crazy part of it all, and I feel weird saying this, was that I was so happy. For the first time in a long time, I felt God providing my spirit with hope, joy, and rest, despite the outcome. This power of hope from God was such a gift! God and His Word changed my prayer life from a "woe is me" type to prayers asking for Him to receive the glory. My deepest yearnings for a child were influenced by Samuel's story from the Bible, where Hannah, Samuel's mom, prayed that if God gave her a child she would dedicate him to the LORD. God changed my heart, changed my worship and prayer life, and now all that was left was for Him to change me physically so that I would bear children, if this was His will.

Infertility was and still is the hardest part of my life, but when I reflect and write this, I am reminded over and over again how God is good, God loves me, and He will provide the peace and joy that sustain me.

UPROOT

What do you turn to when you feel hurt? How do you (if you do) seek aid for your pain?

PLANT

What could be possible if instead of turning to something other than God's presence and provision—in prayer with His Spirit, in His Word, in His family, in His counsel—you took the brave step of believing the promise in Psalm 147:3, that "He heals the brokenhearted and binds up their wounds"?

CHAPTER 3

Till Infertility Do Us Part?

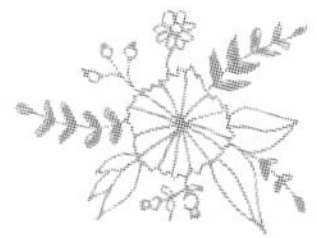

Then Elkanah her husband said to her, "Hannah, why do you weep? Why do you not eat? And why is your heart grieved? Am I not better to you than ten sons?"

—1 SAMUEL 1:8

When we say "I do," we usually say it in the context of a vow to be with each other "in sickness and in health," for "richer or poorer" until death. But these days we know full well that marriages unravel over all sorts of failed expectations. In his book *Preparing for Marriage*, Dennis Rainey begins with an entire section dedicated solely to "Great Expectations." The reason is that no matter what we have in common, what we agree on, or what we are committed to, if we have different expectations on any matter, we will be disappointed. To the degree our expectation mattered, we will be *that* disappointed...even devastated. So the real work in establishing a solid relationship is not just in securing compatibility, but in identifying and addressing expectations up front. Even then, when what we openly hope for and expect to happen *doesn't*, it is a rocky road to travel. A road that is better navigated together watching for God to guide the way. These are some of the expectations Jonathan and I had about children and family before our infertility journey began and how they changed in the process.

Expectations for Children—*He Said*

I grew up in a very connected, hands-on immediate family environment, with large extended family gatherings for holidays and summer vacations. I had one brother and I wanted children, but I never thought in detail about what my family would look like. (However, I did ask God to give me a wife who looked like Pocahontas! He answered that prayer better than I could have imagined.) I just knew that no matter what my family looked like, or how it was made up, I would love and enjoy and want them.

Expectations for Children—*She Said*

I grew up with my parents, one brother, a few cousins nearby, and one set of loving grandparents. But by the time I started working, due to divorce and deaths, my family was reduced to just three, with one grandparent living at a distance. Holidays could get depressing, as I longed for a house full of family bustling about with stories to share. I had always daydreamed about being married and having children—eight to be exact. I'm not sure where that number came from, but entering marriage I desired many children both through pregnancy and adoption. It never occurred to me that I may not have children, but we went through the section on expectations in our premarital book and had that discussion. I remember sitting on the floor of my townhouse, on the phone with Jonathan going over the questions during our courtship. I asked him what he would do if for some reason I could not bear his children. Without skipping a beat he laughed, of all responses! He said, "I'm not marrying your uterus, Heather. I'm marrying you, whatever that means for me." Little did either of us know how this response would serve us as an anchor in our marriage.

Infertility Treatments—*He Said*

I think the hard part about infertility treatments for a man is that it doesn't involve something being done to your body. Instead, it required me to be on my knees a lot before God making sure that I was paying attention and sensing from Him what was needed. I didn't want to subject Heather to undue stress or pressure or surgery unless we both believed God was directing us that way. Another hard part about treatments is the realization that they may work and they may not. With adoption, it was more hopeful that we would be able to parent. The ups and downs and unknowns that come with treatments was something we had to think and pray a lot about. I'll never forget what our doctor said: "No matter how good things look under a microscope, it still takes a miracle to create a life." We believed this, but I believe it more deeply now. It takes a miracle to create a family—whether that's through adoption, infertility treatments, or natural pregnancy.

Infertility Treatments—*She Said*

Since I was on the women's ministry staff at my church, I heard infertility stories surface from many women. I received contact information for local doctors, and listened to dozens of personal stories about various types of procedures. I also heard stories of homeopathic methods, chiropractors who help cure alignment issues blocking pregnancy, acupuncturists who restore blood to the reproductive organs, and of all the ways chemicals make fertility challenging today. To say infertility issues feel overwhelming for a woman is an understatement.

As we consulted infertility specialists and tried to process the information, we decided to start conservatively and I made as many changes to my everyday routine as possible to improve our chances of conceiving naturally. When we chose to start IUI (intra-uterine insemination—traditional artificial insemination where you take medication with a well-timed in-office medical procedure), I was nervous about hormones making me even crazier than I already felt. I was a deep-feeling woman walking through infertility in today's online world! I heard some scary stories from women I knew too, and was aware that countless other stories existed.

We also needed to decide how we were going to bring our struggles into the light. We chose to share our journey with a handful of trusted family and friends (and my boss) so they would be praying for us. I was experiencing one of the losses with infertility immediately: the loss of privacy. Our reproductive journey was public because *not* having kids is a conversation. Doctor visits are with strangers, and grief can hit you in random ways, even in public at social gatherings. We realized we needed to build a support system. Thankfully we made a beautiful discovery in the midst of this loss: community can form like new healed skin around a wound. This treasure in our darkness was really one of so many we would collect on our journey.

The actual treatment itself, though, was not as bad as I anticipated. If the medication made me more emotional, it was hard to tell from my norm. The office visits were something out of the movies—a turkey baster and a dimly lit office with ultrasound machines and assisting nurses. As I quietly focused my eyes on ceiling tiles, my mind would try to balance the tension between hope and grief. Hope for life to form in my body, and grief that it was coming down to this procedure to make it possible. I'd try to scrub from my mind the images of baby bumps pictured in the hallway, trying to not get ahead of myself. Ladies, you know this is a futile exercise. The heart hopes against all odds, and really this is such a healthy thing even though it feels so risky!

After our first IUI treatment, I assumed we would get pregnant right away. Our blood work showed no medical reason why we could not conceive. We did everything the doctor and most infertility books told us to do. I was using natural deodorant that was leaving me a little sweaty by supper. Surely all this obedience would be rewarded, right? On top of that, I started the new hormones the very first day of my new role as women's ministry director. Somewhere secretly in my heart I thought this was the equivalent of me stepping into the river by faith, working in ministry over moms' groups while taking infertility medication. Surely faith and "righteous work" would be rewarded with a pregnancy. Isn't this how it worked? I'm embarrassed to admit just how legalistic I was, and still can be, creating rules and formulas for God to follow in our lives. God was not following any of my rules, though. Our first IUI treatment resulted in no pregnancy.

Surely faith and "righteous work" would be rewarded with a pregnancy. Isn't this how it worked?

After our second IUI treatment, I thought that was our chance. Our doctor had talked about doing up to three rounds of IUI before considering next steps. He didn't want to waste our time, money, or my eggs. But I didn't think God would take three rounds. I fully expected this second one to "work" for us. So when it didn't, I was crushed. I had shed many tears before this point, but this was a lower low for me. It started to dawn on me that bearing children may not be God's plan for us after all, and nothing in me had wanted to embrace this reality until this point. Then to make things even more disheartening, our doctor didn't think a third round was worth the effort. He suspected I had endometriosis that required surgical intervention. With one phone call I learned that I was not pregnant after the second round, and that I would be going in for surgery in a couple of weeks. My surgery would fall two months before a large women's event I was hosting and speaking at, so I would prepare my notes on God's faithfulness while I recovered. Little did I know that this rhythm of writing and speaking in the midst of grief and recovery was also part of God's perfect preparation for me.

Christmas came with its happy songs of a baby in a manger and went with no baby in my womb.

After this kind of surgery women are apparently their most fertile for six months. Again, my hope sprang up with the thought that I'd be pregnant by Christmas (which was the next month). But Christmas came with its happy songs of a baby in a manger and went with no baby in my womb. The women's event came and went too, as did Valentine's Day, and soon spring and Mother's Day with no surprise announcement saying, "We're pregnant!" The conversation then shifted to IVF (in-vitro fertilization—medication with a surgical removal procedure followed up with another surgical procedure), as well as adoption, and I wondered how we got here.

At first I was very nervous about IVF. I knew there were even more hormones involved, spouse-administered shots, more surgical procedures and unknowns for my body, my soul, and our marriage. But after hearing our doctor's team go through the entire process, schedule, and costs, for whatever reason it didn't seem as burdensome as I had imagined it in my head. Jonathan wasn't as overwhelmed as he had imagined either, and we went home with a real decision to make. We had believed it may be our time to adopt, and that this IVF consultation would help affirm that decision, but instead we felt torn with what to do next and set out to seek God's best for us over the next two weeks. We didn't know that when we left that office we would never walk back into it...or see our doctor again. Our treatment journey ended there, and I can say gratefully to God that we have never looked back. God had a plan to grow our family, but it would come about another way.

Adoption—*He Said*

Adoption was never one of those things that I thought about really. I didn't talk about it or think I'd want to adopt children someday. I wasn't exposed to the idea of adoption much growing up, so I just didn't have a lot of forethought or expectations around it. When Heather and I were preparing for marriage and she brought it up as a desire she had, I was fine with it and open to it, but it wasn't something I was passionate about like she was.

Later, though, the more I started thinking about adoption, and what it means that God adopted me into His family, the more my depth for understanding the love of God grew along with my love for Him. I really began to know the love of a Father who chose me, raised me, cares for me as His own, and would even lay down His life for me...because that's what I would do for my child. Then later when it was time for us to decide, God gave me a clear desire of my own to go find my child through adoption.

Adoption—*She Said*

In 2003 I read a book by Randy Alcorn, *Safely Home*, that birthed in me a longing to adopt a child from China. I couldn't explain it—

I had no specific interest in Chinese culture prior to that, or even to adopt, but a strong desire formed in me. I journaled it all out with prayers and wondered how God would do it, because I didn't even have a boyfriend at the time!

I had worked in a law firm during college one summer where adoptions were handled often, and knew the process, the language, the challenges, and the unbelievable joy of seeing families created. I shared my desires with Jonathan early, before we were even engaged, because I knew it would be a challenge in our marriage if we didn't share this vision for our family. Thankfully, he was open to God building our family in different ways, but I prayed even then that if God opened a door for us to build our family through adoption, Jonathan would be more than willing. I wanted him to be filled with joy! God answered those prayers with peace and joy for both of us. Ironically, it would be Jonathan's joy that would buoy me in my own struggles with doubts in later years.

When to Fold Them—*He Said*

Heather has assumed some things about my heart in all of this that just aren't true. For example, she titled this section "When to Fold Them" because she thought I felt there was a time to "throw in the cards" with growing our family. This just isn't the case, but she is keeping the language this way to serve a bigger point: we assume things about each other and are often wrong.

She was right about our journey (which will unfold more in the coming chapters): we have been through a lot. It has taken its toll on our family at times, but I don't see struggles as a sign that we should necessarily quit pursuing children. Our decisions have not been based on our weariness in hard times. Instead I have seen us hold on to a peace because God is sovereign in our family. I believe He has built our family intentionally. I was filled with this peace after we adopted our daughter, knowing that this is the family God built, and it's a miracle. If more children are His plan for us, He can make it abundantly clear for us without us scrambling to "make it happen." I feel sure of Him, more than ever, and so I never need to "fold them" and have never "folded them." Honestly, I probably never will because we will keep on parenting whoever God brings us, until He brings us home.

When to Fold Them—*She Said*

I didn't know how I was going to let go of my dream for children, or later in our journey, for more children. I still long for a big family. Even as I write these words today, years later, I have an empty crib set up in the upstairs guest room just in case God brings us another child. After adopting I hoped that maybe we would get pregnant, or would adopt again. But as our parenting journey continued through fostering, and windows closed for us with adoptions, I started to wonder if maybe God was calling me to accept a different plan for my family.

Finally, one night at my brother's house where we were visiting my newest baby niece, I sank into the guest bed next to Jonathan and felt a peace wash over me like I never had before. I knew our visit would be a test for me. Holding a newborn would either revive my engines to pursue adoption again or would settle me into a restful place. While I did still long for a baby, and in a way always will, I was at peace with our family. I told Jonathan, "I'm good. I'm good with us, the three of us. I think we are good here. This is good. I am good. Let's stop."

With that his chest swelled up like a whale surfacing above the waters, and he released a giant sigh of relief. God answered both of our prayers with peace like a calm river flowing over parched ground. So today we still have a crib in the guest room. It sits filled with stuffed animals and blankets prepared to serve nieces or nephews or friends who visit.

Amendment: After hearing Jonathan's response to this section, I was convicted that my faith is still so small. God is the one who formed life in our family, against all odds. There is no doubt that God conceived our daughter for us through adoption, brought her to full-term, and delivered her into our arms, making her forever ours. If God could do this for us, what else is possible with Him? All the best things for us, that's what.

And all the best things for *you*, too. We never "fold them" when we live with a God who brings life from the dead, and brings children into our families through the most unlikely means. And maybe our crib sits ready for another child . . . if that is God's best for us.

ABRAM SAID | SARAI SAID

I am so grateful for stories in Scripture of real people who make really poor decisions in their pain. Don't get me wrong, I'm inspired by the heroism of faith displayed by so many men and women in our history, but doesn't it bring your soul hope when you see God make space for the ones who really blow it, too? Think about it. What if our wild, unwise, emotionally charged choices made in a moment of desperation are still mysteriously capable of being redeemed by God for His good purpose? This hope was enough to fuel my first book and is often what helps me get out of bed in the morning. It doesn't mean we go headstrong into our days, reckless with our words and decisions because God can still make things good. No. But God has laced the pages of His Word with images of grace in the stories of broken people in pain.

I'm particularly encouraged that God includes intimate insights into the private pain of couples who struggle with infertility, the grief of childless widows, the loss of women who miscarry, the disappointment of women who never marry and those who do but find no joy in it. I've struggled against doubts in God's goodness as I have felt my way through my own disappointments and have found comfort in the tension in these women's stories. God's goodness and our grief are not adversaries, but actually work together to produce godly character in us. When the "happy ending" doesn't turn out for some biblical women the way they dreamed, we see God work in them a dependency and perseverance to know Him. What they find then transforms them forever.

Consider Abram and Sarai, a "He said | She said" of epic accounts. Moses is believed to be the author of the book of Genesis, where the story of Abram and Sarai is found. Personally, I find it interesting that Moses, a man with his own adoption story containing both a Jewish heritage and an Egyptian upbringing, is appointed to describe a Jewish couple seeking a child through the womb of an Egyptian maidservant. Whatever Moses' impression may have been of this couple's motives, we can trust God has sovereignly allowed for the telling of their story in Scripture just as it stands. But it leaves us with so many questions! (I cannot be the only one who reads this story and wants more detail!)

God has laced the pages of His Word with images of grace in the stories of broken people in pain.

Right out of the gate, in Genesis 16:1, we see Moses set up the narrative already leaving gaps: "Now Sarai, Abram's wife, had borne him no children." I read this with an infertility lens and wondered: Did he blame her? How long had they been trying? Was she ever sick? Was he? Were they the only ones in their family to struggle with infertility? Was this something they talked about in the tent at night? What was *that* like? Did wives cry themselves to sleep as husbands snored away? Did she have anyone to talk to among the "flocks and herds and tents"? Did they privately wonder if this was payback for lying to Pharaoh years earlier when Abram said she was his sister? Maybe she thought they would have been bearing children back then if they weren't busy being disobedient to God.

And how does this fit with God's earlier promise that He would give Abram and his "descendants" (literally seed) a huge land to possess and would make them "as the dust of the earth; so that if a man could number the dust of the earth, then [they] also could be numbered"? (You can read this epic baby announcement by God in Genesis 13:14–16.) Sarai must have been so hopeful upon hearing that news. If she was anything like me (prepare yourself for pure speculation), maybe she thought: "I have a man who talks to God, more goods than we can manage easily, and now we are going to have a beautiful homestead with lots of babies! All my dreams are coming true!"

But then something happened. That something was nothing. At least, nothing inside of Sarai's womb for a long, long time.

Years later, we get a brief update when Abram and God are having another one of those vision chats. After God tells Abram not to fear, that He will be his shield and exceedingly great reward, Abram seems exasperated and fainting in hope when he says, "Lord GOD, what will You give me, seeing I go childless…? Look, You have given me no offspring…" (Genesis 15:1–3). God affirms His promise to Abram, adding that the heir will come from his own body, not another form of kinship, and it is recorded that Abram believed God.

However, Sarai isn't present for this promise from God; she only gets the retelling from Abram, a husband who really expected a child! I wonder if she doubted whether God was speaking to Abram, or if the sun and hard labor were getting to him. Did she feel pressure to produce an heir to please her man, her God, and her own longings? Being a woman, I cannot help but believe she did, even in her own unique way.

Moses then goes on to introduce Sarai's maidservant, an Egyptian slave named Hagar. From what we can see of Sarai's emotional state during this season, she seemed to be struggling to trust in the God who gave her husband promises and visions. Sarai points straight at God for why she hasn't had a baby yet and pulls the trump card with Abram for why her plan to have Hagar bear them a child is the way to go: "See now, *the LORD* has restrained me from bearing children" (Genesis 16:2). For some the excuse may be, "The devil made me do it," but for Sarai it was, "The LORD made me do it"! She felt justified, believing the LORD gave her no choice but to take her future into her own hands.

Despite God's law regarding marriage, that a man leave his father and mother and be joined to his wife so they become one flesh (Genesis 2:24), Sarai concocted a plan to "obtain children" through Hagar's temporary union with Abram. This form of surrogacy is fraught with problems, as you can imagine. Before we peek into the problems they created, I'd like to pause to capture a couple of helpful lessons from this plan of our sister's: 1) we are wise to seek counsel before we make decisions that impact our home life, and 2) when we feel desperate, rather than devise a plan, perhaps we should take a walk among the trees... because God tends to speak to people, like both Abram and Hagar, in that space.

Now the event escalates until we can almost hear the narration shift from Moses to Abram and Sarai sitting at a table recounting the disaster after the fact. Would you allow me some creative license to consider what our ancestors may have said? Some day we will get the true story, but for now imagine what could have happened in this scene:

Abram: God promised I'd have an heir.

Sarai: Yeah, I heard you the first time. That's what I was trying to help make happen because it wasn't working the old-fashioned way, remember?

Abram: Well, I wasn't telling you it had to be this month!

Sarai: Umm, every month for years your face said it all!

Abram: What was I suppose to do? Act like I wasn't disappointed?

Sarai: Well, I was trying everything I knew how. Do you think I wanted the word "barren" in my story? No!

Abram: I didn't say this was your fault, I was just telling you what God said.

Sarai: Well, He never told me. He hasn't even talked to me. I felt like I was letting you and God down every time you shared one of your "visions" with me.

Abram: I can't help it if you don't talk to God for yourself; that's between you and Him. I'm not God, Sarai, I'm just telling you what He said. Don't shoot the messenger!

Sarai: Well, it's not like attempting with Hagar was illegal or something. Everyone is doing it. I wasn't in the wrong there.

Abram: No, I never said it was illegal.

(Neither of them even mentioned the whole issue of God's law for marriage established with Adam and Eve.)

Sarai: Well, you definitely didn't hesitate to cooperate with my plan, that's for sure!

Abram: You made me! What was I supposed to say? You said, "Please," and had been so upset for so long! I just wanted a happy wife for once, and maybe that was what God meant by giving me an "heir"? I didn't know what would happen either!

Sarai: Well, a giant mess, that's what happened! For one, it broke my heart that she conceived. It confirmed my fears—I'm the reason we don't have children. Then the heartache with Hagar knocked my knees out! Here I tried to run a peaceful home and trusted Hagar, and all I wanted was to have an heir—just one heir! You would think after knowing us for over a decade, knowing my longing for a child and my struggle, that she would have shown me a little compassion when she got pregnant!

Abram: Sarai, it's what you wanted, though, right? A baby? That's all we heard!

Sarai: Yes, but not in strife and pain. She despised me after she found out she was expecting. I was worthless in her eyes, mocked. She rubbed it in my face and hated me for it at the same time. I couldn't handle having her baby bump and words jabbing at me all day. If I was wrong, then let my wrong be upon you! Let the LORD show who is to blame here!

Abram: Fine. I'm out. You do what you want, you always do anyway.

Sarai: Fine. I will!

(Both go separate directions, slamming tent flaps as hard as it is possible.)

CHOOSING THE HOPE OF THE COVENANT

The one word that helped hold Jonathan and I together when infertility threatened to rock our marital boat is this: *covenant*. Knowing that we were called to each other, to marriage, with God in our union, helped us lean into each other rather than fall away. We weren't sure God was calling us to bear children, but we knew He had called us into the covenant of marriage. Covenants are not contracts that can be breached due to a party's failure to perform. A covenant is a binding agreement to honor a promise regardless of the other party's performance! In other words, nothing can separate you from the hope of that promise being fulfilled.

For Abram, God's promise was sure and was not dependent on Abram and Sarai's ability to produce a child or live faithfully to God. God was just going to be faithful to Abram, period. In our marriage, knowing that Jonathan was going to love and enjoy me as his wife, regardless of whether I bore him heirs (and vice versa), helped us embrace decisions united rather than divided. Like Isaac prayed for Rebekah to conceive (Genesis 25:21), Jonathan would continue to offer comfort to my grieving heart but led our family to hope in God for what was best for us.

In the story of Abram and Sarai, God not only viewed their marriage union as sacred, but He made a covenant with Abram, binding Himself to a promise to Abram's descendants (Genesis 15:18). More than fourteen years later God reaffirmed this covenant with Abram.

But what of Sarai? We see Abram talking with God, getting visions that stirred up his hope of heirs, while Sarai is unmentioned, perhaps grieving somewhere in her barrenness. Had God rejected Sarai for her disobedient rush to make her dreams come true? What about her blame-shifting to everyone else for her pain? We'll talk more about her story later, but there is hope for Sarai, and there is hope for all of us who do things in our desperation.

Hannah's Story

From the beginning of our marriage, nearly every decision my husband and I made was in anticipation of growing our family. We planned down to the month when we would conceive and naively rescheduled a cruise as I would then be "too pregnant" to travel. Nine months later, instead of welcoming a baby into our home (as seemingly everyone around us was doing), we were blindsided with the diagnosis of unexplained infertility. Suddenly we were dealing with feelings of shock, depression, jealousy, and worthlessness, as well as the loss of privacy in the most intimate part of our marriage. I began to believe that not being blessed with a child meant that we had actually been cursed, and so I settled into the pit of infertility and covered myself with the blanket of self-pity.

I was comfortable wallowing for far too long. Although it is natural and important to work through the stages of grief, I allowed my anger to become habit-forming and my jealousy to become consuming. It is hard to admit that as a "mature Christian" my identity was partially built on self-ability. Unsurprisingly, that foundation quickly crumbled in the face of childlessness. I know that season caused my husband a lot of pain as he tried to support someone who was determined to just lay down; but, by the grace of God our marriage survived and was strengthened as the Holy Spirit patiently nudged me into a healthier perspective.

This new perspective involved releasing my plans into the hands of Someone who had not only the desire but the ability to work all things together for good. I often prayed, "Lord, in my desire to be a mom, please do not let me step outside of Your will. Give us wisdom, peace, obedience, and contentment in every circumstance." Instead of focusing on what was missing from our lives, I began to intentionally look for and name my blessings.

It is fitting that I share a part of my story alongside the story of my infertile sister Sarai. I intimately understand the desire to make my own plans, to right the ship, and to provide a child for my husband in the face of infertility. The Holy Spirit, through several unique situations, began to challenge me with this thought, though: "This year might be the last good year you have with your husband, and you are wasting it grieving a changed future." I began to look around and realized that, while I felt left behind by all of my peers, in reality I too was blessed beyond measure. Even in the midst of infertility, God had a plan and was at work. Now I look back at my younger self, who in naive anticipation rescheduled a cruise for no reason, and I feel a little dread for her. She had no idea about the heartbreak that was just around the corner. It was not a pleasant journey, in fact, it was horrible. But there is joy on the other side. As God graciously gave Sarai a new name, He has given me a new perspective and an identity built firmly on His truths and not on my plans.

UPROOT

What is one belief about marriage, or your spouse, that is hindering you from being united?

PLANT

What does God say about that belief?

CHAPTER 4

The Decision to Adopt

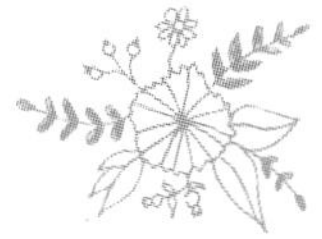

So Hagar bore…
whom Hagar bore…
when Hagar bore…

—GENESIS 16:15,16

When I practiced adoption law in Florida (2004–2006), I was moved by the powerful adoption imagery God uses in Scripture. I marveled at realizing I am His child by adoption, through saving faith in Jesus Christ. It was during this season one night when I found myself reckoning with my own sin tendencies, wrestling with the dead weight of shame. I made my way to a park near my house after work, and settled in at a swing set. As I curled my legs under me and stretched them out to fuel my pendulum, I confessed how distant I felt from God, how unlike Him I looked. My heart was weary with immaturity and I wondered if God felt the same way toward me. In the gentlest way, though, He seemed to cup my heart in His hands and whisper, "You are Mine. I adopted you, Heather. You don't necessarily look like Me because of this, but wait. The more you spend time with Me, and learn from Me, and enjoy My love for you...you will start to take after Me. In time, the highest compliment anyone will ever pay you is that *you look just like your Father!* And you will, child of Mine. You will!"

My soul took flight with my feet. I flew clear off my seat mid-swing into the dirt, but I didn't mind. Delight spilled out of me as I took in the realization that God saw me as His child, dearly loved. It mattered not that I didn't really resemble Him yet. I was chosen through adoption, hand-selected to be His own, and that gave me all the dignity and worth I could ever hope for, and we would simply grow together from there.

Not all adoption stories ring so sweetly, though, at least at first. I witnessed adoption stories in my life that were hard to understand. Stories where couples who could not conceive brought home beautiful babies only to have to return them to birthparents who changed their minds. While working in a law firm that practiced adoption law, I watched the lead attorney drive to a home with a car seat to retrieve a precious little bundle from a completely wrecked couple. Their loss of a dream was met with another loss of a baby they were able to hold in their arms for only a few short days. That experience shaped me with its lack of answers, and decades later I would return to that scene playing out in my own life, with me asking God for understanding once again.

A TIME TO BE SILENT

When Jonathan and I set out on our adoption journey, we were both all-in. In hindsight, we see God's hands all over our need for assurance that this was His plan for our family, because it took all the grit of faith we had to make it through intact. We had already endured infertility treatments, and after surgery for endometriosis I went another five months without conceiving before our doctor said he'd like to talk about next steps. Time is precious in fertility matters, so he didn't want to waste our time on measures that were not likely to work for us. Since I was nearly thirty-six years old, he suggested we move right into IVF efforts. We appreciated his zeal and early in April 2013 we set appointments for an IVF consult as well as an adoption meeting with an agency, for later that month.

You can imagine how the topic of bearing children dominated our conversation for months. The strain was starting to wear on both of us. I was continuing to work as women's ministry leader at our church and Jonathan was managing and preparing to take ownership of the only thing growing in our family—a family business. Neither of us knew what direction God was leading us to choose for our family. We had more questions than certainties with every path. What we did know was that God had called us to the covenant of marriage, and we wanted this to be our first priority. No matter what we decided to do *about* our family, we wanted to do it *as* a family, united. So with what we now see as God-inspired wisdom, we committed to taking a break from the discussion of children to just breathe and be together for a time.

Two weeks, to be exact.

We decided that for two weeks that April we would take the topic of IVF and adoption off the table, and would instead talk about every other thing, or nothing at all. You can imagine how awkward this was at times, being such a huge elephant in every room. But we knew that this was where we needed to begin with our commitment to our marriage. We knew that if we let "our kids" get between us before they were even born, it would be that much easier to let it happen in the future. So we went on dates, we held hands during movies, we snuggled on the couch, we prayed and talked about dreams, work, health...and let the issue of our children sit under wraps with God.

During those two weeks, though, God allowed for the most bizarre and interesting conversations with other people. Every single day of those two weeks, whether I was in the car, or in a meeting, or in a store checkout line, I was brought into a random conversation about adoption. Completely unprovoked, and even with my best efforts to be left out! After a full week of it, I wanted so badly to tell Jonathan and make sense of it, but the topic was off limits. So I waited, and the daily unexpected nudges toward adoption continued. It helped that Jonathan was away for most of that second week at a remote location in Arkansas with no cell reception. (I think God knew I couldn't keep quiet, and helped us honor our commitment by preventing our communication. Smooth, right?)

When Jonathan came home from that trip, minutes dragged on as I helped him unpack. He had just finished a twelve-hour car ride, so the last thing he needed was to be drawn into a deeply emotional conversation. (I am still learning this discernment, so don't be fooled by this momentary lapse into maturity!) Honestly, I was a little afraid that what I had to share could serve to manipulate or persuade him to agree to something that was outside of his personal desire. More than anything, I wanted us to be aligned in joy, so we could move out with peace in whichever direction we chose together. But in a few moments all my concerns would fall away, because what we had to share with each other was nothing short of divine direction.

Every day of Jonathan's two-week break, God nudged him with some conversation on adoption—even on the White River in Arkansas, in a boat between two friends he thought he knew well. There he was quietly enjoying the peaceful serenity of nature and manly bonding over fishing, when his buddy in the front of the boat (an empty nester) turned to show him a picture on his phone of his new son in Haiti. They would be traveling to meet him later that year. Jonathan was stunned. This was the very last thing he expected to hear from this man. Then his buddy in the back of the boat chimed in, "Man, that is awesome! Ya'll don't know this about me, but I was adopted." It's a wonder my man didn't faint and tumble right over the edge of the boat. He said to me, "Heather, I don't know God's plans for our family but I know two things: 1) God has called us to parent, and 2) adoption is no longer a question, it's time to set out."

God was helping two clueless people recognize the good path He was putting before us. We knew right then, on a sunny afternoon in April 2013, that we were launching out on our adoption journey. I hopped in the shower after our morning talk and began sobbing loudly with joy. To assure Jonathan I wasn't upset, I yelled through the shower door, "I feel like we just got news we are expecting!" He yelled back, "It's because we are, baby!" What we didn't realize was that in that same month God conceived our daughter in a womb not that far away.

THE THINGS PEOPLE SAY

You hear it from people all the time: "Oh, you can't have children? Have you considered adoption?" Can we officially delete this line from humanity's verbal bank? I would bet money I don't have on this statement: every couple who has ever struggled to conceive has considered adoption. Of course they consider it, how can they not? Adoption is incredibly beautiful in its life-giving exchange, but in order to give life there is always pain, tearing, labor, and loss of some kind. As with much of life, the sacrifice is worth it (we would walk out our journey a thousand times over again just to be who we are today, have what we have today, and know what we know today)—but it is important to check expectations at the start because there is much at stake in this journey, for many people. When couples consider adoption, it is (and needs to be) a deeply complex and personal journey.

First, suggesting adoption to couples struggling to conceive presumes that infertility grief is easily addressed by the presence of any baby at all. If you didn't know this before now, let me make something plain: *adoption does not cure infertility grief.* Gratitude doesn't displace grief, either. We can be deeply grateful for good gifts and blessings in our lives, and yet grieve the loss of dreams at the same time. Adopting, fostering, and birthing children are unique journeys that bring with them unique challenges and blessings. The better we understand what they involve, and accept that our expectations may need to adjust, the better we can move forward in a hopeful way.

Our lives with their blend of bruise and blessing, with God, are gifts chosen by Him.

I heard people say to me, "I know it's not your Plan A, but adoption is such a beautiful choice." I struggled with this for a long while, and my theology explained why. We all move toward dreams and plans based on our desires: relationships, degrees, jobs, and so on. We don't always end up with the things we pursue, though. And this isn't a bad thing, if we trust our lives to God! We are always becoming the people God intends for us to be, in the joys and the hardships. I personally believe infertility and adoption were always God's Plan A for us. God has all knowledge, over all history, so it is impossible for Him to be surprised by failed infertility treatments. Yes, God created a perfect earth with perfect humans who could procreate and live forever. Yes, He intended for us to live in unending peace that was broken when Adam and Eve chose to sin. Yes, God cursed the earth as a result, and as creatures dependent on the land this means we feel the impact of that curse in our bodies.

But even there, in the Garden, God saw our family story completed. He saw how far the curse would ripple into the future, and how it would impact our family. Just as His move toward humanity was in love and restoration through animal hides, He made a way for our little family in the beginning, too. God designed a Plan A for us to experience His goodness and restorative love today, and wove a redemptive purpose into our pain.

We are not manufacturer defects that He needs to be alerted of, or that need to be recalled. No. Suffering in this life is also in Plan A for us. We were surprised, yes, but not God. Our family dynamic, childless couples, single women, or widows are not living in some Plan B life, settling for God's leftovers. I don't want to make light of pain, loss, and disappointments, but I actually believe that *this* is our best life. Our lives with their blend of bruise and blessing, with God, are gifts chosen by Him. Believing this, we can hold onto hope that by His grace we can live meaningful lives and deeply enjoy them too.

Some other statements that may hurt a woman with an infertility story include, "We want more children but don't want to go through another pregnancy." Yes, some women suffer near death in delivery. That path is not easy either. (Is any path easy, really?) But this statement can gong in the ears of women with infertility because again, choosing to build your family or "have more children" is a luxury not all enjoy in this life. Even for women able to conceive, they may be nursing grief due to divorce, abandonment, loss of provision, or loss of health. Many women who have an infertility story long for more children but are unable to grow their families through adoption for one reason or another (like finances, or emotional limits that keep them from extending themselves into more complex relational dynamics).

On the other end of the spectrum are the prideful boasts of how easy it is to bear children. I have heard, "All my husband has to do is look at me and I get pregnant," or "We wanted our kids to be this far apart, so we picked just the right month to conceive our next child and made it happen!" I remember seeing a very pregnant woman wearing a shirt that read "I make babies, what do you make?" It took God, Jesus, and His Holy Spirit to hold me still and not do the two things I wanted to do: 1) bawl my eyes out, and 2) give her a good tongue-lashing for being so insensitive to a good portion of women who will never have that experience.

Then there is the comment that is not intended to give offense or put women with infertility on edge, but can be hard to swallow: "We really want a little (girl/boy) from (foreign country) to *complete* our family." I understand wanting more children. I do, I desire it as well. I understand feeling like something about your life doesn't yet feel complete, stepping out to discover what that is, and finding it's another child. I have friends who have birthed children, then felt God calling them to find their other children on foreign lands. They don't distinguish or wear their kids on their sleeves like trinkets that make them "cool" families—they were sincerely obedient, led by the love of God, sacrificed in labor, and were all-in as parents ready to go the distance for "their child."

But this isn't the case for all families, unfortunately. I have heard comments from some that still makes the hair on the back of my neck stand on end. Cases where the desire was more to create an idyllic multi-national Christmas card than to lock oneself on to the well-being and nurture of a tiny human with a world of hurt in their story. Again we see that, like with Sarai, when we rush ahead to "make ourselves" what we long for rather than seek God for His provision and path, we may instead find that we make ourselves a mess.

THE OTHER WOMAN

Adoption stories are complicated by nature. You are folding people into your family who are unrelated to you, but who hold biological ties to your children. When you bring an infertility story into this dynamic, it can get even more complex, because the one thing you wanted to do (birth a child) is being done through another woman and man. I don't care how mature you are emotionally, or spiritually, this dynamic can just be tough at times. As elated as I was to see our daughter's image on an ultrasound, it pierced my heart to be in a room where my belly wasn't the one being examined, and never could.

I've also noticed a recurring pattern in mothers with an infertility story, based on my experience with dozens and dozens of adoptive families. The dynamic of engaging with a birthmother who is biologically related to their child can be more sensitive for them than for women who can bear children. In fact, some of my most confusing wounds have come from conversations with women who have both adopted children and birthed children, talking about their relationships with the birthmothers. Perhaps it is their shared bond in giving birth to children, but generally speaking I have observed an ease in their ability to relate to birthmothers. Mothers of biological children seem to have a more natural empathy for birthmothers wanting a connection with the child, and seem less threatened by "sharing space" with her.

Even if it is a healthy dynamic for everyone involved, hearing stories like these can make a woman with an infertility story feel shame for not being able to connect better in this way, or "share space" without feeling insecure or threatened in her role as the child's mother.

Distinguishing children by categories, such as "my adopted children" versus "children of my own," is problematic for several reasons, too, and can be especially hurtful to mothers with an infertility story. For one, the distinction dishonors your child through adoption as "less than" yours. I understand what is meant by that statement: one child is not biologically related, and the others are biologically related. While this is helpful information for your pediatrician, I don't think it's necessary or helpful in everyday introductions. Mothers with an infertility story don't generally falter on this line because we could not bear our child biologically. By God's wild grace this is our child. The judge looked us in the eyes at our final hearing and said these words: "Now this child is yours, as if she came from you biologically—forever yours." Where she was born, and under what biological circumstances, are for her to care about and her doctor to know. Otherwise, this is just my child, end of story. After our final hearing, when it comes to who the mother of our child is, the answer is simply *me*.

In cases where women have adopted children, I notice this element just in different degrees: a struggle with security in one's identity as a mother. If a woman bears children biologically, I find that she is most secure in her identity as a mother. (I'm not talking about confidence in *being* a mother, mind you!) No one questions this security, this connection, or her role as "mother." It is highly honored, celebrated, and even guarded by the law unless extreme reasons demand otherwise. This security remains with her as she adds children to her family through adoption, even though birthmothers are connected to her children.

But when you cannot bear your children, there is still a thread of insecurity in your role as mother. First, there is no distinction, no labeling of your children, because they are *all* yours thanks to God and the law. And yet, this woman can feel vulnerable and unsure of her role as mother, because of the birthmother who stakes a kind of claim on her child, too. Just like for Sarai and Hagar, there is something you don't bring to your mother/child dynamic: you didn't birth your child. The other woman, even if not physically present in your family dynamic, is always there in your story and in your relationship with your child. So terms like "their *real* mother" can feel like an even deeper cut to a woman with infertility. She is reminded of her closed womb and is left to doubt if she will ever "really" be considered a mother.

WHAT TO EXPECT WHEN YOU'RE EXPECTING *IN ADOPTION*

I said it before, every story is unique—and this is especially true with adoption stories. I will not even pretend to speak for every family, because that would be impossible. However, I will share from what our community of adoptive families have experienced, which is a fairly sizable group. Surprisingly, the community is largely represented by couples with an infertility story too, so I feel like the themes I share in this book are legitimate—not just because it is our personal experience, but because it has been shared by so many with similar situations.

After Jonathan and I decided to start on our adoption journey, we met with an agency and were drawn to both the international adoption track and domestic adoption. We had no clear leaning either way, but were drawn to the program for children in China with minor and correctable special needs, as well as to children in our region. After research, prayer, and counsel, we learned we could do both tracks simultaneously. Our home study would serve for both tracks, and our domestic home study would simply be the first half of the paperwork required to pursue a child internationally. In all of our meetings it was clear to us we would most likely travel to China first, because we were fairly open to conditions that were prevalent in children waiting for families. We were told it was even possible we could travel to China within a year after all our paperwork was finalized. Alternatively, the wait list for children in our region extended long enough to last a couple of years.

Hope was brimming and I was ecstatic and yet also afraid of the impending disappointment.

So when Jonathan and I submitted our completed home study and picture books in in November 2013, we left for the Bahamas to celebrate our five-year anniversary and believed there was no way we could bring home a child for at least two more years. It was a bittersweet trip for me, too, that I'll share more about later. For now I'll just say that God sees us, cares about our hearts, and is in the business of showing off for us sometimes in ways that can only be explained by grace.

When we got home from our trip, we returned to work and routines and I began the international dossier paperwork. But just four days after being home, we received a call from our adoption agency. When I saw the number I first thought we were getting the call that our home study was approved! I was trembling with excitement at the thought.

"Hello?"

"Hello, is this Heather?"

"Yes! Hi!"

"Hey, Heather, we wanted to ask if you and Jonathan are open to having your profile shown to a birthmother this week?"

Silence. Choke.

"There must be some mistake. We haven't even had our home study approved yet."

"Oh, wait a minute. Thank you. Someone will be in touch with you soon."

I hung up and my heart sank at the thought of possibly being considered, then it being wrong. Then the phone rang again—it was the adoption agency.

"Hi, Heather?"

It was a different voice this time.

"Yes?"

"We have good news! Your home study has been approved!"

"Oh, wonderful! We are so thrilled!" I imagined we had gotten the call earlier by accident. It was probably meant for a family above ours on the list. I tried to shake off the lingering disappointment and chose to embrace excitement that we were now officially able to start the rest of the application that would take us months to complete.

"*And*...we are wanting to know if you and Jonathan are open to having your family profile shared with a birthmother this week?"

Silence. I couldn't even find my throat to choke.

They explained why we were being considered so soon, that the dynamic just fit us better than most and that we would still be one of three profiles shared that week.

"Yes. Absolutely. Yes!!!"

When I hung up, I could think of nothing else but that phone call. I called Jonathan shaking, crying, already coming up with all the reasons this would probably not be our child...*but, what if?* Hope was brimming and I was ecstatic and yet also afraid of the impending disappointment. I went back to the church where I worked for a meeting with my supervising pastor, and shared the news. He prayed with me and we talked about what this might mean for our ministry plans. If I were to bring a baby home that year, I'd need margin to adjust. (How little did I know how true this would be for us!) Even as we spoke, I could hardly believe the words coming out of my mouth.

The next few days passed with no phone call, and we assumed we were not the family picked. For three days I denied it bothered me, but on the fourth day my driveway found me doubled over, sobbing. No one really knew we were hopeful, so no one really knew we were sorrowful. It was the strangest grief, like a loss no one could see or touch. We had plenty to do to keep us busy through the weekend, but by that next Monday I was sick at home with a cold, letting the sadness mingle and release with the congestion I was blowing out of my nose.

Then my phone rang.

It was the adoption agency.

They had been very busy, but... we were the first ones picked!

I don't remember feeling sick anymore after that, and called Jonathan to rearrange his schedule because we were needed there the next day to get more of the story and to make our decision to proceed.

I'm saving the details of our meetings, and of our times with the birthparents over those next couple of months, to share with our daughter. She knows some of these stories already, and loves to hear them. But I will share that we had the fullness of joy that Christmas of expecting our little girl, of knowing her name, of seeing her wiggle on an ultrasound, and had plans to watch her enter our world later in January 2014.

Please understand that this is just one story. Many couples, including ones we know well, wait months, even years, to meet their children. And some never get that call. Not only is pregnancy a miracle of God, but as my husband says, "It takes a miracle to create a family." And even when an adoption door does open, this is just one of several hurdles you need to clear before welcoming your child home. For couples with an infertility story, this emotional minefield can be even more painful, because at each stage you remember that you aren't the one pregnant. You aren't the one who gets to decide what happens to the child that may be yours, not in the beginning. If your focus is on wanting a child, your pain will be acute. But if your focus is on the God who has your family in His hands, trusting that He is sovereign and gives you the challenges and blessings that are *good* for you, then the adoption journey becomes your front-row seat on an adventure where you continually witness God's power play out.

ERRING ON THE SIDE OF LOVE

Jonathan and I were ecstatic. We had made plans to be in the delivery room to welcome our daughter into the world with the help of induction. We traveled to the city the day before and settled into our hotel wondering how we would sleep a wink. We ate a meal and learned the waiter had been adopted, and he spoke of his love for his parents. He brought us a slice of key lime pie with a candle in it to celebrate her birthday, and we laughed. I remarked that it was a day early, but we'd celebrate all the same.

It could have been the sugar crash from the pie, but we fell into a deep sleep that night, only to wake to a call we weren't expecting. Our daughter had been born earlier that day, but we had all been cut out. We had missed her birth, and were faced with the reality of losing her altogether. We were stunned. We had nothing to point to for a warning sign. However, we knew the statistics. Families roughly have a 50 percent chance of making it to the delivery of their child. Then those families face a new hurdle where they only have a 50 percent chance of actually making it out of the hospital with their child. Even then, those parents only have a 50 percent chance of making it through the hearing terminating parental rights, which is separate and necessary before moving to the final adoption hearing. This means families have a high chance of grieving the loss of their child through adoption—because when you hear news that you are expecting a child, for all intents and purposes you *are* expecting a child.

The call came like a gut punch. Our little girl was breathing our air, and we weren't there holding her. My chest crushed in on itself from crying so hard. I didn't know whether to go ahead and grieve our loss of her then, or maintain hope. Our agency wasn't sure what to tell us either. A birthparent was straddling the fence. We were told to just stay at our hotel and not leave the city and that they would keep us posted.

For sixteen hours we stayed numb in our hotel, with me crying in waves like contractions. We ordered in food we barely ate. Then finally we received a call to come in for a meeting at the agency. It didn't sound good. We learned there was still a chance the adoption plan would continue forward, but the agency recommended an interim family placement since it was such a high-risk adoption. The thought of our daughter going to an interim family made us ill. We had built trust with the birthparents and I didn't want them feeling like strangers would be caring for our girl—as wonderful as I'm sure they would be. We decided that this was our child no matter what. If she was placed with a family, it would be in ours. If we needed to return her, we would be the ones to bear that pain and would grieve the loss of our daughter.

I remembered the story of a friend of mine who had carried her sweet baby girl all the way to term, only learning toward the end that she was not going to survive. She had forty-five minutes with that beautiful baby girl of hers. I reasoned, *Who am I to have any longer with my little girl?* We made plans to stay in the city, awaiting a hopeful word that we could at least see our girl for forty-five minutes. And of course, we prayed with all we had in us to have her much longer.

Finally, two days later we were invited to the hospital and checked out of our hotel. Regardless of how our visit ended, we would be going home that night. We walked into a hospital room that became the holiest ground I've ever stood upon. When we looked into the eyes of our daughter and then held her, we were undone. We later heard that the first words said of our little girl at birth were, "She looks like Jonathan and Heather." What grace. And it was true! She was our delight from the first on-screen wiggle, and here we were getting to see the fullness of a child God seeded in our hearts... maybe for such a time as this.

We prayed over her privately for a few moments. I used her name and told her we loved her. I prayed she would know Jesus and His wide love for her. I prayed that she would grow into the beautiful woman God designed her to be, and that she would always know how much we love her. Even in that room we felt the 50 percent chance of raising her, and of losing her, swinging us from hope to heartache. As our conversation moved along, the plan seemed to shift with each sentence. But we had decided to go to the hospital room to show love, no matter what, and it was proving to be a sacrifice of love beyond what either of us could have imagined. God gave us a desire to actually err on the side of love, and see them, see our girl, speak life to them, pray with them, and offer them grace. Jesus was with us, giving us what we didn't have in us to give. It flowed from a grace and peace He gave us the night before in our hotel room.

Finally, though, the time came for us to go sit in the waiting room as a placement decision needed to be made. We still hoped that we would be taking our little one home with us. After all, why would we have been given such peace and love for this long? Surely this was God's plan for us? But God's plans sometimes come through closed doors as well as closed wombs. I'll never forget the sight through the windows veiled by partially closed horizontal mini-blinds. Our social worker was making his way to us slowly, with his head drooping like a man on his way to tell parents their child was gone. Seeing our jackets and bags in his arms, I knew. It was time for us to go home. Alone.

God's plans sometimes come through closed doors as well as closed wombs.

Many women know the grief of a miscarriage. While I do not know *that* pain, I imagine the emotions are indescribable and disorienting as you try to make your feet walk out of a hospital with arms empty. Jonathan gripped me tightly against his body as we stepped out of the elevator and headed toward double glass doors that opened so easily for us. It seemed ironic that some doors do open so easily, while others never budge. I felt his fingers dig into my arms as the blizzard wind blistered against our faces. I don't know if it was to keep me upright, or him. We said no words and I bit my lip until I was inside our car with the door shut.

With no emotion released at all I simply said, "Let me text everyone so it's all done and I can turn off my phone." He started the car. Words stumbled through my fingers and I shut my phone down. I couldn't handle anyone else's sadness but ours in that car ride. And ours was about to come out in full force.

I have put this part of the story off for weeks because I didn't want to relive it. Even today, it has felt like labor pushes that lead to no baby. I write a paragraph, take a pause to release tears, and feel tired because I'm not done yet. I wonder if this section on humanity will ever end. And so I feel the groans of our earth, waiting on the coming of Christ to fully redeem all our tears for joy. Some days we can just take one paragraph at a time.

As Jonathan pulled out of the hospital parking lot and hit the highway, with my phone put away and nothing but grief and road ahead of us, we both lost it. I think the only thing more painful than crying my own heart out was hearing my man cry his out. There was nothing I could do to fix his pain, nothing he could do to fix mine. We were faithful to what God asked of us; we went to our finish line, but it didn't feel like a celebration. Instead of fireworks there was fire in our hearts burning up our dreams before our eyes. At the same time, though, we had peace in that fire. We knew God was with us. There was no doubt we had experienced His presence in the hotel and hospital rooms. He was with us in the car, even though we felt numb and ordered food through a drive-thru window like this was the most normal thing and we weren't about to wail for another five miles of road. We knew He was helping us drive, even though it was taking us several hours with pull-offs to wipe our eyes to see. Just a few exits away we chose to trust that He would help us walk into our home, and her room all decorated, as well.

Then Jonathan's phone rang.

We got news that we could go back and get our baby.

You know the classic movie scene when the husband is driving the car like a maniac to the hospital, while the pregnant wife is beside herself screaming, moaning, crying, and occasionally saying, "I love you, baby, I'm sorry for being so crazy. But, drive faster!" Well, that was us. I turned my phone back on to call my mom, Jonathan called his dad, and we asked for everyone to get on their knees.

A couple of wild and bittersweet hours later, we were in a new hospital room alone holding our daughter. *Our daughter.* Jonathan fed her a bottle for the first time. I wept. She slept in my arms while we signed a thousand papers and watched videos from the 1970s on newborn care. I spoke briefly on the phone with a birthparent and the words were some of the most intimate words I will forever hold close. I relive those words when I need hope.

We drove home slowly and with abundant joy this time, with me snuggled as close as I could get to our littlest bundle of sheer grace. She was hands-down the most beautiful baby we have yet to lay our eyes on. We were drunk with gratitude, our words stumbled into giggles of praise to God for surprising us in the midst of our grief. We arrived late that night back at our home filled with our family to welcome our girl home, and of course, we barely slept the entire weekend and didn't mind it at all.

NOTHING IS FINAL UNTIL IT'S FINAL

Remember those statistics I referenced earlier? We cleared the first 50 percent chance of getting to the delivery, sort of. Then we cleared the 50 percent chance of taking our child home from the hospital, barely. Now we had our other 50 percent chance of making it through the termination of parental rights hearing. What we didn't realize that weekend, while we were lavishing kisses and prayers and songs on our daughter, was how fragile our little family still was at that time. The Monday after our sweetest weekend ever, we received a call from our adoption agency. We needed to take our daughter back. We were facing the 50 percent chance of loss head-on.

To be clear, we knew this was a high-risk case, and that choosing to place children with families is the hardest decision of a person's life. We had built relationships with some of the people in our daughter's story, and our hearts broke deeply for them. We wanted them to have a good life too. Adoption just creates these moments that are incredibly complex and painful, as well as overwhelmingly good and filled with grace and love. So I don't share this making light of suffering. No. I can only imagine the pain of letting a child go, which I did get to taste that month as we held our little girl and then moved to give her back.

We hung up the phone and the three of us sat on our couch, crying, holding each other, willing ourselves to get up and go pack up all of her stuff and make the long drive back to our agency to say good-bye to our daughter. Again.

At some point over the next hour as we packed, my phone buzzed. We learned we were allowed to keep our daughter. I thought for a moment that I was losing my mind; the relief swept in as fast as the grief just an hour earlier. This time, though, I remained guarded. The buzz of my phone set off an immediate reaction of nausea in my stomach and adrenaline surged through my body moving me to anxious tears. I was afraid to enjoy the sweetness of our daughter. I felt hostage to constant shifts of will that I was powerless to prepare for or prevent. We asked our agency to only use Jonathan's phone number. I needed to shut my phone off.

Day by day for several weeks we engaged in tense talks with people who influenced the future of our family. We were constantly aware that our time with our daughter could end in one moment. With each mention of "if not" we faced a reality that we may still grieve the loss of our daughter. Since we didn't know how long we had with her, we brought friends and family into our home to pray over us, pray over her, and just be with us. We savored every moment. We sang to her, we kissed her until her skin could take no more. We drank deeply of the goodness of God in our little family and realized how precious a gift it truly is to welcome a child into the world.

I'll wrap up this story now with a quick finish, because you may need some relief from this emotionally winding story, like I do! We did make it through the hearing to terminate parental rights, against all odds and to the surprise of our adoption agency even. Ironically, it was the same day her little umbilical cord fell off, as if her body was severing the connection to embrace a new one. Six months later, we stood before a judge at our final hearing and heard the most beautiful words: *It is final.*

Apart from God, we can do nothing. But with God, even the barren can be mothers.

I cannot help but think about the relief we have as Christians to similar words spoken by Christ on His cross: It is finished. All the heartache, the sacrifice, the blood shed, the payment for an old life so a new life can be born, is found complete in the cross. Jesus chose us and paid for us to be adopted by God. God accepted His offering, and then was the Judge who issued the decree recognizing us as His own, with a new name and new future.

See, adoption is not about getting babies. It is about trusting God to give us what is best for us as we are utterly and completely dependent on His provision and timing. It is true for our eternal salvation, for our families, and for every other thing we face in this life. I spoke about security earlier, for women in their roles as mothers. My security in being God's daughter does not rest in my ability to be a good Christian woman. My security as a child of

God is sealed up in God's final judgment based on Jesus' petition and payment for my life. Ultimately, too, with regard to my infertility story and desire to be a mother, what I came to learn (and am still learning) is that our security as mothers needs to come not from our children at all, because in human terms we just may not get them in this life. Our security as mothers comes from the One who *calls us all to motherhood.*

All women who trust Jesus with their lives are adopted daughters of God. Our lives are no longer our own—we belong to Him. None of us are entitled to what we have today; we are only entitled to a hope in Christ to redeem all things for our good and God's glory. My daughter is my daughter. But in a way, she is not. This is not because of adoption, but because God is God. She belongs ultimately to God, as do I, as do you and yours. Infertility just provides clarity for us, reminding us that we don't really have the power to create life on our own. Not really. Apart from God, we can do nothing. But with God, even the barren can be mothers.

And He is calling all of us, His daughters, to motherhood.

Regardless of what your womb, or agencies, or birthparents say, we are created to be *mothers*—ones who raise up others—in this generation.

Tabitha's Story

My husband, Thomas, and I met in the summer of 2001, and I knew by November that he was the man for me. We talked about a lot of the important things couples talk about before getting married and knew we wanted to have kids, sooner than later. When we married, I was already twenty-nine, and he was thirty-one years old, so we didn't want to wait very long before trying to start our family. We had both wanted two kids. We had grown up that way so it was what we were familiar with and what we imagined for our family. So after a year of being married, we decided to stop preventing pregnancy and tried to start growing our family.

After a year of not conceiving, we talked with the doctors. They ran tests and said they didn't understand why we weren't getting pregnant. Everything on our tests said we were healthy, just not conceiving. We started infertility treatments confident that would work. We ended up going through four IUI treatments and then two IVF rounds, and they didn't work. We saw beautiful embryos transferred, and watched them on the ultrasound, but then lost them eight to ten days afterward. It was horrible. We took pictures of them, and still love them as our babies. I couldn't understand why my body wouldn't work. If the doctors couldn't explain it, and it was the desire of my heart, why were those babies not staying there? I was an early childhood major even, and thought this was God's plan for me. I remember the day I got the letter from the doctor. It was a list of everything that had been done, and an explanation that there was nothing else they could do for us. It was awful. That was when I really experienced anger. Anger toward everyone, especially God.

Even now I cannot hold back the tears, remembering how awful the pain felt, how dark it all was back then. I wouldn't wish it on anybody. I was so mad at God, there were six months when I wouldn't talk to Him. I didn't go to church. I isolated myself from everyone who loved me and grew depressed. My husband stayed by my side, but his way of handling the pain was different and didn't help me process my own grief.

One day, I woke early and just took off driving. I had been depressed for a while, and between my own emotions and pain, and his responses with anger and blame at the doctors, I just needed space. So I grabbed our dog and drove to a beach out of town. I checked into a bed & breakfast. I didn't call in to work or call my husband. Later I knew I was insensitive to not let him know where I was going, but I was so heartbroken and weary of it all, I just needed to be quiet. I did later call my husband to assure him I was okay, that I just needed to get away a bit. But that's how rough things had gotten, for me and for us. He was having a hard time understanding what I was feeling, and I wasn't helping him because I didn't know how to communicate what all was going on inside of me either.

Also during this season, my sister was pregnant. There were showers back in my hometown for her, but I just couldn't go. Later, during that Christmas when we were visiting, a cousin chose to announce her pregnancy to everyone. It was the straw that broke the camel's back for me. After everyone left and my husband went to bed, I fell apart in my parent's kitchen. Nobody understood. My parents came around me and squeezed me so tight as I sobbed. We all cried for forty-five minutes as my mom simply prayed over and over through her tears: "God, we don't understand, but we're trusting You." It was a hard night, but I felt something in that moment, too. The pain didn't go away, but there was a small peace growing in me that helped me to believe somehow it would be okay.

After we returned home we were ready to pursue adoption. We also received counseling by an infertility specialist who helped us communicate our feelings with each other. Having a third party really helped our marriage. We weren't able to afford both the fertility treatments and adoption expenses at the same time, so we began saving for the adoption. Before we married, we had talked about adoption though we didn't really know why. We were both open to it, but "our plan" was to have one or two children biologically first, and then maybe adopt a child. We didn't know a lot about adoption, though. Growing up, we each knew maybe one family with an adoption story, but people didn't talk about it much, not like we do today.

As we started researching different agencies, we kept hearing about one local agency in particular and would see signs for them. It felt like God was directing us to contact them, so we did. They provided classes for us to attend, so we did that too, and initially we felt like we could handle only a closed adoption. We had already been through so much disappointment and loss, we just felt guarded. We imagined sitting in our home with our child to hear a knock on the door from biological relatives wanting to take our child or ask for things. After finishing our classes, though, we were willing to consider a semi-open adoption.

Our adoption process took four years. We even moved during our wait time, but our agency agreed to keep working with us since we had already paid so much money and been waiting so long. It was so hard. We said we trusted that God had a plan for our lives, but I don't think I really believed it. There was a song on the Christian radio station at the time by John Waller, with the lyrics, "While I'm waiting, I will worship," and I sang it maybe a million times every day. Somewhere in this season I had a heart change and surrendered to God that He *did* actually have a plan for our lives! We were heading into another holiday season and my husband and I both went from just saying the words, "We trust God," to truly believing He was trustworthy! I got to the place where I said, "Lord, whatever You want. I know You are in charge, and You know the desires of my heart." This time, though, I really believed it.

We light-heartedly talked about how we were going to be that couple who travels the world and does the coolest things. I had a nephew who was just a great kid, and we talked about enjoying him as much as we could. When we were back in my parents' home for Thanksgiving, as we were enjoying our family, we got the call from our agency. We had been picked, and were expecting a daughter! Three years after standing in that same kitchen crying in my parents' arms, with my mom proclaiming a trust I couldn't proclaim boldly myself, we stood together again this time crying tears of joy!

We met our baby girl in 2009. Six years of heartbreak and loss, confusion and anger, became our trail of tears that turned into trust. We trusted God knew what was best for us before we met our girl, but it ended up being better than we could have imagined. We were able to enjoy an organically healthy relationship with our daughter's biological connections, and even moved into an open relationship we still enjoy today. Where we had fears over expenses, God provided everything we needed.

Three years later, we wondered if God had a plan for us to be a family of four or stay a family of three. We knew this time to trust God had a plan for us, and not to be worried over it, so we contacted the agency again, this time in another state. We decided to do a home study for just one year. If God planned for us to have another child, we believed it would happen that year. If not, we would be okay with that ending. A few months before our home study was set to expire, I got a call from our agency while at work. We were shocked to learn we would be expecting a little boy! We consider him our extra special blessing from God for our family, because we know how unusual it is for a family to grow that fast through adoption.

To anyone reading, I can tell you that it's one thing to say God has a perfect plan for your life, but another to truly believe it, and live like you believe it. That is what made the difference for me. So now when I'm struggling with something or we are going through a hard time, I truly have no doubt that we will get through it and will be better for it somehow. I truly believe God has a perfect plan for my life. To not believe this would be so awful. I know because I was there. I cannot imagine living any longer without this true peace in trusting that God is who He is and is faithful.

Thomas' Story
(Tabitha's husband)

When Tabitha was depressed and hurting, I felt helpless. I wanted to blame someone, anyone, and chose the doctors. I cursed and yelled about their incompetence and wanted to get other opinions. I just didn't know what else to do. It hurt me seeing her so broken, and honestly, I didn't know if she'd ever come out of it. I was afraid it would last forever. Later, when we started the adoption process, I was still nervous. I was afraid of more heartache and of her sliding back into depression. Even when we got the call that we were expecting, I felt guarded. I wanted to be excited, but I also saw her excitement and knew she would be devastated if this didn't work out for us.

I wasn't as strong in my faith then as I am today, so it was hard for me to trust God with my family. Even in the delivery room, I felt afraid of something going wrong, like years earlier when we would see the babies on the ultrasound, then lose them. I didn't think our hearts could handle losing another baby. Thankfully, back then the law was only forty-eight hours before you were in the clear, no longer in danger of having the adoption plan fail. I knew she could see the relief in me; it was like I was finally able to breathe. I knew it was safe to love my baby girl, and that was the easiest part of all.

UPROOT

What belief do you have about adoption that is hindering you from either saying "yes" to it or "no" to it this season?

PLANT

What does God say about that belief?

CHAPTER 5

A Time to Weep

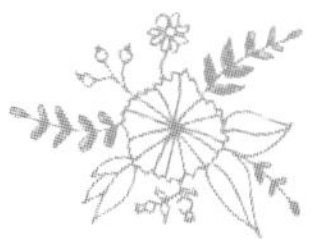

To everything there is a season, a time for every purpose under heaven... a time to weep, and a time to laugh; a time to mourn, and a time to dance.

—ECCLESIASTES 3:1,4

When we are in the midst of a season, it is challenging to process what we believe about God, ourselves, and our circumstances within that season. Often it takes time to understand what has settled into our hearts from the storms and hurts we endure. During this processing, if we courageously choose to allow it, we may discover emotions we didn't know we were capable of feeling. In fact, the fear of being overwhelmed by the discomforting feelings related to our pain is often what keeps us from feeling them in the first place. If you listen to me long you hear me say this: it is not unhealthy to feel negative emotions—it is unhealthy to *never* feel them. The unavoidable truth is that pain refuses to be avoided forever. In time, the body sends out signals through the gut, the spine, the chest, even the skin telling us something is off within. Signs may show up in other places, too. It may be relationships fracturing, bank accounts bottoming out, or, like me, it could be pants demanding more space that finally serves as a wakeup call. No matter the form of the warning, the pain is the same invitation to join God for a time to weep.

BIG GIRLS AND BOYS *DO* CRY

For some reason, many of us feel shame for weeping. Even privately, we shame ourselves for getting "so emotional" as if it were a design flaw to express emotion through tears. We apologize for doing it in public, excusing it as just our hormones, claiming we haven't slept enough, or saying we're being overly dramatic. No wonder it is so difficult for men to express emotions with tears; women denounce it as a weakness of our design. It seems strange to think of feeling "bad" about crying considering that we never feel shame for using the bathroom! Or for sweating, or spitting out what tastes bad, or even throwing up (which I have done publicly and yes, have apologized for…but still, I felt compassion toward myself in that moment and received the compassion of others).

So what is it about crying that makes us so self-conscious? For one, we feel incredibly vulnerable in that it exposes our heart. We see all our other bodily releases as physical and natural; those responses do not risk revealing our innermost feelings, hopes, or fears. We don't feel bad about doing what we are simply designed to do; there is no shame in being a person physically. We feel bad, though, about being *our* person. We feel bad for thinking our thoughts and feeling our feelings. This is perhaps God's enemy's finest use of shame: making us believe we are wrong to think, to feel, and to be the fully human beings God created us in His image to be.

So we need to set the record straight: God is for weeping. He made it part of our design, a mechanism by which we release honest emotions that express our innermost longings. Grief is not something to avoid, it is a gift to help our fully human being heal and repair. Like with other physical responses, we build up emotion within and must release it regularly in some way. Ideally, we will give ourselves compassion and room to express it in ways that are dignified and healthy, without shame. Otherwise, the emotion will find another way out that may make things much more difficult, both for us and those around us.

For women with an infertility story, and for any woman who feels barren of soul—where you feel like you have nothing to offer—there is a time to weep over what is a real loss of some kind. In the next chapter we'll talk about where dreams go when they die, because there is a death we eventually accept with infertility, or whenever something we deeply long for goes away. But in this chapter, I want to shape the way we see weeping, and offer a hopeful mindset that refreshes rather than weighs down. After all, God would not give us eyes that weep unless He had a very good reason.

HOW WEEPING SERVES US

In the recordings of the prophet Jeremiah, God confronts the disobedience of the people He created: "But they have walked according to the dictates of their own hearts and after the Baals, which their fathers taught them" (Jeremiah 9:14). The consequences are not favorable for Israel, but God gives them instruction on what to do to move toward restoration:

> "Consider and call for the mourning women, that they may come; and send for skillful wailing women, that they may come. Let them make haste and take up a wailing for us, that our eyes may run with tears, and our eyelids gush with water." (Jeremiah 9:17,18)

This doesn't sound like God shames weeping. Far from it. Weeping was a holy and appropriate sacrifice to bring for the sin and shame of a disobedient people. The prayer of weeping women mourning over the loss of peace expressed the grief of God. Women could even become "skilled" at mourning, praying out grief over sin and shame according to the will of God. And so great would be the need for mourners, the mothers were encouraged to teach their daughters to lament (Jeremiah 9:20).

While this passage was in the context of Israel's rebellion, we live in a constant culture of rebellion against and rejection of God. Our bodies and souls are exposed daily to the dark side of humanity and the consequences of a cursed earth. The good news is that we have the joy of Christ's victory over both sin and shame through His sacrificial death on the cross. And yet, as He redeems the curse through His Word, His Spirit, and His Church, there is an appropriate response to pain in our world today. Even more so, there is a healthy response to the pain in *our* worlds. We have the gift of weeping as a form of expression of the grief of God for suffering, and a real release for our own.

Another way weeping serves us is that it can be communal. One of the reasons we feel shame for weeping is that we feel shame for appearing weak. Our culture values power and strength, not vulnerability. We base success on the person we beat rather than the person we become. We confuse fame for worth and meaning, and so we build versions of ourselves to display when our souls get pressed with a need to weep. But this is not God's design for our souls, or for success. Jesus was clearly the most powerful person on the planet, for no ruler or king has ever defeated death itself. His power was limitless and yet He restrained Himself for the purpose of fulfilling God's will for His life. He welcomed His humanity as a gift to connect with us. And Scripture tells us that Jesus wept. He even wept publicly. Jesus can identify with our broken hearts because He is "a Man of sorrows and acquainted with grief" (Isaiah 53:3).

How overwhelmingly loving for the God of all creation, with unlimited strength and ability, to humble Himself to our human frame with human emotions and human expression that could be misunderstood and mocked. And what did He weep over? Before a crowd in the town of Bethany, He wept after seeing His friend Mary weeping along with other Jews grieving the death of her brother Lazarus. Jesus knew Lazarus had died, and knew He was about to bring him back to life. He may have been weeping over the lack of faith of His friends, that those who knew Him still doubted He was the all-powerful Messiah. Or, maybe He wept out of compassion for those grieving, feeling their pain as His own—because we *are* His own.

Jesus also wept as He drew near the city of Jerusalem, its residents hustling about preparing for Passover completely blinded to the fact that the Messiah was making His triumphal entry on a colt.

> "If you had known, even you, especially in this your day, the things that make for your peace! But now they are hidden from your eyes. For days will come upon you when your enemies will build an embankment around you, surround you and close you in on every side, and level you, and your children within you, to the ground; and they will not leave in you one stone upon another, because you did not know the time of your visitation." (Luke 19:41–44)

We miss Jesus every day. We miss His entrance into our small stories. We call it something else: luck, or good fortune. Then we feel overwhelmed and brought to the ground by the challenges of our day, all because we aren't looking for Jesus. I wonder if in these moments He weeps. Not so much because He feels forgotten by us, or undervalued. He always knows who He is and can never feel belittled. But I wonder if He grieves our loss, the sadness for what we are missing out on by looking at the gods of this world rather than the World-maker.

Weeping also helps us become who we are meant to be, and invites others into who they are meant to be as well. When we weep we make room for our limits, our hopes, our longings, and our fears. Over time, connecting with our emotions before God and one another, we grow in understanding ourselves, our needs, and God's heart for us. We invite others to come close to our hearts to be strong for us when we feel weak. This is less about transferring power to another person than it is recognizing each other's power. I have power when I weep because I am choosing to be vulnerable, which is enormously brave and costly.

When we weep we make room for our limits, our hopes, our longings, and our fears.

When someone chooses to share that space with me, they bring their own power of listening, of choosing to be vulnerable by feeling their humanity in order to connect. This too is brave and costly. Many of us know the awkward sense of rejection when we cry and others seem to be uncomfortable, distant, with a "what's wrong with you?" look on their face. Weeping without shame and within community is a practice, so no wonder God asks the women to train their daughters. We can pave the way by bravely weeping over our grief, so they feel less vulnerable bringing their tears.

Weeping is also good for our bodies. Psychiatrist Dr. Judith Orloff shares research explaining how emotional tears have special health benefits:

> After studying the composition of tears, Dr. Frey found that emotional tears shed these [stress] hormones and other toxins which accumulate during stress. Additional studies also suggest that crying stimulates the production of endorphins, our body's natural pain killer and "feel-good" hormones.[5]

Could it be that the gift we offer the next generation of women is the permission to grieve? What could happen to the statistics on teen suicide, on depression and anxiety, if we answered the instruction of God to train up and call out the wailing women? I want my daughter and the women around me to know that weeping is not only human, it is spiritual. It is designed in them for their physical release, as well as for the soul's well-being, and honors the God who made them.

Weeping sometimes helps push new life out that would otherwise stay stuck within. In a physical sense, this is easy to see. In childbirth, women bear down and cry out, laboring and wailing as they bring new life into the world. But the soul works in a similar way as we experience the new life of Christ being born in us. We travail through the burning off of pride and shedding of self that comes with the conviction of sin. We mourn the depravity of our desires, the blackness of our heart. We weep over the inability to purify ourselves, to make ourselves clean before a holy God. And in the death of our flesh, we find the sunrise of a new day, a new story, a new hope where mourning ends and joy ushers in through mercy. In the sacrifice of weeping, we sow seed that brings a harvest of joy and fruit into our lives! Listen to the benefit hidden in weeping here:

> He who goes out weeping, bearing the seed for sowing, shall come home with shouts of joy, bringing his sheaves with him. (Psalm 126:6, ESV)

I hope you are beginning to see weeping in a new light, that weeping with someone is powerful. To sincerely cry over the loss of a loved one, a season, or a dream is to say they or it mattered. It declares to the world that this beautiful gift of God existed once. It has dignity and touched your heart in such a meaningful way that the absence of it is now felt deeply. It was desired, wanted, treasured, and is now missed. We speak worth over one another, honor the gift in one another, and show love for one another when we weep.

WHEN I FINALLY WEPT

As I've confessed, I tend to avoid feeling negative emotions. I love laughing and fun, dancing and playing, entertainment and comfort. But there is a time for everything. There is a time for some things to end so others can begin. Like feeling the pain that builds up in our souls.

While I felt sad about our inability to conceive early on, and cried tears, I didn't fully weep and mourn our infertility for years. During our season of infertility treatments, it took all my mental and emotional energy to stay hopeful and not drown in a million tears. Without realizing it, I began carrying a weight of appearing to be "okay" in front of Jonathan and friends, so as to not add to his burden or suck all the oxygen out of every room. In my private moments with God in my living room or out walking on our farm, I would feel the surge of emotion well up within my chest so intense, I feared my heart would burst. We have only a few neighbors on our country road, so thankfully the days when I would double over on our driveway in heaves of grief were still just between God and I. Even with those occasional outbursts, though, it wasn't really until years after we brought our little girl home from the hospital that I began processing the reality of infertility and what it meant for my family.

I can say from my journey that if you don't have a Christian counselor to process your grief with, or a community of women who are growing in emotional health with Jesus and understand your grief, pray for one. Go online and/or call your local church until you find one. I was working in women's ministry when we were processing infertility, infertility treatments, adoption, and then post-adoptive trauma (which I'll share more on later). I was not seeking counseling at the time, because I thought my time in God's Word, in prayer, and in worship and service at my church was giving me all the strength I needed.

However, warning signs in my body and my soul were telling another story. I was struggling with anxiety, shortness of breath, and chest pains. I felt a constant self-imposed pressure to be everything to every woman who emailed, called, stopped in, or asked for appointments. I felt responsible to know all the influencers in Christian women's culture, read all the books, know all the challenges facing women, and facilitate the finest small groups and events. As much as I talked about grace, I was oppressed by the need to please others and deliver perfection. Work was becoming an unhealthy escape from the real pain I wasn't feeling. When I got still, I was overcome by fears of what could happen to our daughter. I wondered when we would "lose her" again.

My stomach flipped inside out every time my phone would ding, wondering when a hostile text would come through against me or my family. When my husband started to talk in a serious tone, my heart would race wild bracing for news of the latest verbal attack against us at his work or online. I didn't know it because I wasn't feeling it, but I was as angry as fire is hot over the fact that my daughter didn't come from my womb. I resented some of the painful dynamics in my story that were permanent. I also felt unrelenting guilt for not being able to help people I cared about to heal. I felt guilt for feeling sad when I had such a beautiful family. Then I also felt guilt for feeling happy that I had such a beautiful family. Meanwhile, I was overeating to calm the anxiety, then exercising excessively or depriving myself severely to counter the effects of weight gain. I was in a shame cycle, but didn't see it because I was afraid to feel my pain and weep.

Finally, though, God called out this wailing woman.

My husband and I were interested in seeking God together for His will for our family in terms of limits and protections. We were not doing well with our open relationship in our adoption, and we needed to do what was best for our family. One of the things we decided to do as a couple was to seek God and discern His purpose for our lives as a family. We used a variety of resources for discerning God's will, including His Word and prayer and conversations with others. It was beautiful journey, too. The process naturally required me to slow down and connect with my dreams, which meant I would have to feel things.

In order to get to the joy of dreaming again, I needed to go through the valley of weeping first.

Golda Meir, former Prime Minister of Israel, said in an interview one time, "Those who don't know how to weep with their whole heart don't know how to laugh either."[6] In order to get to the joy of dreaming again, I needed to go through the valley of weeping first. If not for my hope of joy on the other side, I might not have put my toe in the waters, but I did. I soon discovered there was more to it than I realized, so much in fact that I needed to pull back and make space for healing and restoration. Less than a year later I resigned from my ministry position and was at home, on the phone with a counselor for post-adoptive trauma, weeping like I never had before.

You'd think that with the tears shed up to this point my well would have been dry. Think again. I continued for the next two years at home, learning to weep and receive the healing community of Jesus, my husband, and others. I didn't just weep, though. I got involved with ministering to others, including through storytelling as an Ambassador with Noonday Collection. As an Ambassador I get to share stories with others about women and men rising out of poverty through the dignified work of creating handmade accessories I can sell in my community. I found that in sharing their stories, and my own, and extending my soul for their sakes, God was bringing me my own healing.

> "If you extend your soul to the hungry and satisfy the afflicted soul, then your light shall dawn in the darkness, and your darkness shall be as the noonday." (Isaiah 58:10)

God was teaching me how to mourn and to heal by sharing stories with others. When we invite others into our grief, we can better walk out of it with them. Feeling my pain gave me the tools to come alongside other women with new authenticity and power in vulnerability because I knew intimately what it was like to feel pain and walk through it one step at a time. I also knew I couldn't fix anything for them, but could point them to the One who wept with them too.

I will practice weeping for the rest of my life. While life itself will continue to bring with it trials and challenges, infertility grief is a strange grief that never fully ends. More healing for me came, ironically, when I read this verse:

> There are three things that are never satisfied, four never say, "Enough!": the grave, *the barren womb*, the earth that is not

satisfied with water—and the fire never says, "Enough!" (Proverbs 30:15,16)

It dawned on me that God designed women, to some degree, to want to have babies. Not every woman feels this maybe, but the barren womb wants to be satisfied, by design. We want to live on, we want to give life, we want to reproduce meaning into our world. My weeping would come at unexpected times and catch me off guard, even today. At age forty-one and with a vision for what my life is for apart from bearing children, I can still get surprised by my weeping. It helps me to know that God made me this way, that there is a reason I still find myself grieving. A barren womb is never fully satisfied. It doesn't mean I don't enjoy satisfaction, because I do! I'm incredibly content with my life. But again, gratitude doesn't displace grief. Grief is mysterious and rolls in like a tide when sometimes it makes no sense.

We want to live on, we want to give life, we want to reproduce meaning into our world.

As I learned to weep with my whole heart, I realized the truth behind Golda Meir's words. I found a new well for laughter with my whole heart, too. I was able to rest in my role as my daughter's Mama, as my husband's wife, and even found a freer way to yield my voice to Jesus in the ministry to women's hearts. Just over two years after resigning from my ministry position, after two years of weeping in the basement of my home where I learned to laugh again, God opened a door for me to publish a book. It was beyond my ability to comprehend, and every doubt you can imagine flooded into my head. But I know now that God was in the resignation and the book contract. There is a time to weep, and a time to laugh; a time to be silent, and a time to speak.

THE HOPE WE HAVE WHEN WE WEEP

Maybe it will help you embrace your time of weeping if you keep the hope you have with weeping before you.

Remember, we don't weep alone. If you don't believe anyone else weeps, which would be an unreasonable belief by the way, you at least have proof in this book that *I* do. And often! We are in the community of weepers of the highest pedigree, though, including Jesus! Hannah wept. Jacob wept. Jesus' mother wept. Martha and Mary wept. Peter wept. The children of Israel wept. Jeremiah wept (a lot, it would seem). Job and his friends wept. David wept. Solomon wept. Esther wept.

Kings and queens wept.

The God of all creation wept.

We enter into our full identity as image-bearers when we embrace a time to weep. And there is more good news: we won't weep forever.

> Weeping may endure for a night, but joy comes in the morning. (Psalm 30:5)

God moves in weeping, but He also soon moves us out into joy. He knows the flow of our tears, friends, their start and their end. They matter to Him. David seemed to know a secret, that God collects our tears in His bottle (Psalm 56:8) just as He collects our names in His book of Life when we put our faith in Christ.

In this life we will have weeping, but take heart, we will soon have joy unspeakable, too. We can move into weeping, as women who are preparing for harvest. With every brave turn we make with our whole hearts into the presence of our God, in our hurts, we can look forward to the fruitfulness our offering of tears can bring about in God's time. Read this verse again, but let's personalize it a bit because in it is the hope for the barren, that we too can be revolutionaries, bringing about tremendous change in our world:

> Those barren ones who sow in tears shall reap in joy. She who continually goes forth weeping, *bearing seed* for sowing, shall doubtless come again with rejoicing, bringing her children with her. (Psalm 126:5,6, personalization added)

Brittany's Story

I didn't always want to be a mother. Then while I was single and still in college, I was rocking a screaming toddler to sleep for a friend. When he finally closed his eyes I noticed my reflection in the mirror. I thought, *This is what I want out of life. I want to rock babies to sleep. I want to be a mother.*

Over the next two years I met and married my husband. I was twenty-three and he was twenty-five. We both knew we wanted a big family, and I couldn't wait to be a young mom and imagined how we would share our huge surprise like people do on Facebook! So shortly after our wedding, we ditched the birth control and braced ourselves for what we knew would change our lives forever. Except, that moment of excitement never came. We tried to believe that when the timing was right, God would bless our family with children. We tried to move on with hope that this season was our "meantime" before our family would grow.

So in the *meantime*, we started new jobs and bought a fixer-upper home. Then around our fourth year of marriage we decided we were going to "take this pregnancy thing seriously." I bought the whole starter kit: the basal thermometer, prenatal vitamins, and the best OPKs (ovulation predictor kits) you could get. Fast forward two years: after two procedures, multiple rounds of fertility drugs, countless doctor visits and blood tests, it turns out we have a double infertility factor (both my husband

and I are diagnosed with infertility). I was by myself in the doctor's office when I got the news, and my first reaction was shock. I remember the doctor's sympathetic facial expression as he told me the best and probably only option for us to conceive was through IVF (in-vitro fertilization).

After the initial shock wore off, I walked to the billing office. A very sweet woman told me about special financing for IVF. *But wait, there's only a 45 percent chance it will work?* But my chances increase after every round? And each round can cost up to $15,000? I remember holding back tears as the emotions started to come. I walked to my car and wept. Not for very long though; the reality of what we were facing hadn't really sunk in yet. That was only three months ago, and I find myself still in the season of mourning. I am mourning my idea of what life was "supposed" to look like. Mourning children who were "supposed to come" five years ago. Mourning biological children we may never have.

I am angry, resentful, and hurting in ways I never thought the heart could hurt. There have been countless days and nights when I find myself losing control, in the fetal position on my living room floor screaming at God: *"Why?"* And yet, I am seeing how our God is so good, too. It has been in my mourning where He has met me. He sees me. He sees my heart and He holds on to me tightly. Through this trial, I have been learning how to take care of my heart, because the Lord cares so much for me.

I am learning it is okay to not go to baby showers. It is okay to say "no" to working in children's ministry and to skip family functions where everyone will ask when we are going to have children. It is okay to say "no"! Some of my most healing moments for my heart and soul have been at home on a Sunday morning just weeping, pleading, and lamenting to the Lord. I don't know why the Lord chose this path for me and my husband, nor how long this season of mourning will last, but I will cling to Him as tightly as I can as we walk and weep together.

UPROOT

What are you believing about grief and weeping that is hindering you from experiencing deeper peace?

PLANT

How does understanding God's design for us to weep, and knowing what Scripture shows us about those who wept, shape your belief?

CHAPTER 6

Where Dreams Go When They Die

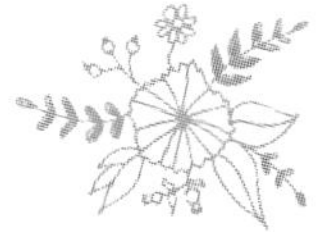

"I say to you, unless a grain of wheat falls into the earth and dies, it remains alone; but if it dies, it bears much fruit."

—JOHN 12:24 (ESV)

My daughter and I talk a lot these days about dying. You may think this is a morbid conversation to have with a four-year-old, but for us it is the most cheerful discussion! She likes to say, "Mommy, when I'm all done growing, Jesus will come get me and take me to Heaven because He forgave my sins already." It is music to my ears to hear the gospel ringing hope in her heart. She's right, too. All it takes for us to be saved by Jesus forever is to hear the gospel and believe it: that Jesus died for our sins, was buried, and raised from the dead three days later. If you don't believe me, believe Paul, who met the resurrected Christ himself after an epic career of being the first official persecutor of Christians:

> I declare to you the gospel…: that Christ died for our sins according to the Scriptures, and that He was buried, and that He rose again the third day according to the Scriptures. (1 Corinthians 15:1,3,4)

> In Him you also trusted, after you heard the word of truth, the gospel of your salvation; in whom also, having believed, you were sealed with the Holy Spirit of promise. (Ephesians 1:13)

With her question settled on where she will go when she is "all done growing," all we have left to do now is our work assigned by God as we enjoy daydreaming with Him. We imagine and talk about all the beaches, ponds, warm bread with salted butter, and animals we'll see in Heaven. She also likes to talk about whether she will have her beloved Pinky Bear (a well-loved teddy bear) with her there or not.

It is a cheerful conversation because the reality of Heaven brings such joy in the midst of days when headlines sink your heart to the bottom of the sea. It seems that every time we turn the television on, or open a news app, another story of death or disease or destruction greets us in the reality of this life. If our gaze hovers here for long, all hope of goodness and peace just drain right out of our souls. We need constant reminders that this is not our Home. This is our place of work. In a way, we are living out a long workweek of sorts, with refreshing work breaks. We will finish our work, because Jesus will see to it; but we are not yet where we can enjoy the deep rest and comfort that comes with being safe and sound at Home. Oh, we get tastes of it, glimpses of what this will be like. We savor these moments and feel the glorious hint of Heaven. But mostly, we encourage one another to stay the course. We choose daily to be all-in where God has us, as we look forward to where our hope will be fulfilled in epic grandeur.

WORKING FROM PARADISE

As a writer and speaker, I do my work in all sorts of places. Often I'm sitting at a farmhouse table in my basement, with piles stacked up edge to edge. But today I'm typing these words from paradise. No, I mean really, it is paradise! We are celebrating our ten-year anniversary in the Bahamas, at an all-inclusive resort on Great Exuma Island. You hate me right now, I know. For the record, we return home tomorrow where there is snow. But here, the Bahama breezes are constant, gentle, and refreshing. Our pace has been slow, without agenda, simple, quiet, still, relaxed, all the things we love in a retreat. And the irony that I am writing *this* chapter, on *this* shore, is not lost on me.

This same resort is where we celebrated our five-year anniversary. It's very easy for us to remember, and not just because we laid still as downed trees for five days then too. It was also the trip I had imagined would be our "baby moon" after our infertility treatments. I had pictured myself here, with full belly, excited to return home and prepare for a delivery. As God would have it, though, this was not our story. We were directed down the path of adoption and had just submitted our home study application prior to the trip. As grateful as I was for clarity and the hope of a child someday, it still felt so far off. We were celebrating within the tension of grief mingled with joy. What we didn't know then, that we know now, was that we were just two months away from welcoming our little baby girl into our world after all!

Originally, for this ten-year anniversary trip, I had no intention of working on this book. I knew this was going to be a deep work, and imagined this trip as a rest from that work. My wise friend said of this book, "Heather, you will leave flesh on the page with this one." Chapters 4 through 6 are skin pages, for sure. I had wanted them done by now, but even last month was too soon for me. I have met with a counseling friend, almost one session per chapter, and several sessions had to pass before I could consider beginning chapter 4.

I shared with Jonathan about my writing wall. He said, "Heather, those are heavy chapters to feel for you. Maybe God doesn't want you to write them from the basement. Maybe God wants you to write them from paradise. Maybe you just need to bring your computer and write on our trip... at the beach."

He was right. This time I have once again left tears in the powder sands of this Bahamian shore, but they have been full of gratitude and healing.

Writing from paradise produces a different work. My perspective is higher, longer, wider, and full of peace, joy, and light. The frame for our stories, and these chapters, is now with the long view of eternity, of blue skies and emerald waters, of bodies relaxed on easy shores. I'm reminded of the perfection that is coming, and the God who knows our dreams (Psalm 20:4), who set eternity in our hearts (Ecclesiastes 3:11), and works all things together for our good and His purpose (Romans 8:28). I relax as I remember He is continuing the good work He started in each of us (Philippians 1:6). In a mysterious way, the conversation that felt heavy before has been made light by the hope of eternity, with a God who makes all things new.

ALL THINGS NEW

As adopted children of God in Christ, when we die (or are "all done growing") we go to paradise. Since this book is not about the theology of our end-of-life experience, I won't go too far into the details of what this will be like for us. Also, I have more questions than answers! But what we know is that when we are done in these bodies, we will be present with Jesus who is making all things new:

> We are confident, yes, well pleased rather to be absent from the body and to be present with the Lord. (2 Corinthians 5:8)

> Then He who sat on the throne said, "Behold, I make all things new." And He said to me, "Write, for these words are true and faithful." (Revelation 21:5)

If Jesus can make all things new, what *all* does *all* include? He makes our bodies new, our souls new, He makes the earth new, He makes the oceans, animals, food, cities, and government new. If we loved it here, if it was good here, if it gave us joy and hope and a taste of His character here on a corrupt earth, how much more can we look forward to enjoying it in a perfect Heaven where *all* things are new?

Maybe even the dreams we longed for here—the dreams of love and marriage, children and family, health and peace, goodness and joy—are *all* made new for us in the resurrection of *all* the things coming soon, too! But even though the hope of seeing our dreams fulfilled in Heaven is wonderful, if we are honest, it doesn't make it hurt any less when our dreams die here in this life.

Letting go of a dream, or a desire, is one of the most painful losses, because what we are desiring or dreaming of gives us hope for tomorrow in the midst of suffering. When our dreams die, our hope for tomorrow seems to be buried with them.

That dream for a marriage we were hoping for... dies.
That dream for a child we were hoping for... dies.
That dream for a home we were hoping for... dies.
That dream of a new business we were hoping for... dies.
That dream of healing we were hoping for... dies.

In our shared humanity, we understand the disorienting grief death brings, so we honor the loss with ceremony, with somber reflection, with mourning clothing, with tears and tissues, and we bring words of love and memories of life to comfort the hearts of those grieving, including our own. But what about when the dream that died was not seen, known, or experienced by others? What if it was contained within the walls of our hearts? What if it was the longing itself that can no longer live? What if our desire is not compatible with life on this earth? What ceremony fits this loss, what clothing, what words of love and memories of life bring comfort to the heart suffering the loss of a dream no one can enter into with us... but God? And how do we reconcile these deaths with God, alongside verses like these:

As all seed and creation experiences, there is no fruit without first a death.

> May He grant you your heart's desire and fulfill all your plans! (Psalm 20:4, ESV)

> Delight yourself also in the LORD, and He shall give you the desires of your heart. (Psalm 37:4)

We are children of a God who simply does not get disoriented by death, or anything else. For God, the passage from life to death is like Monday to Tuesday. There is no change in His view, really. Our souls remain with Him from one space to the other. And so while we are fully human and naturally bent on grieving what we cannot have in this life, our aim is to see our dreams as God sees them. God sees our hearts, and has placed desires in them Himself, knitting them into our being for His special and mysterious purpose. There is no dream we can have that is good, apart from His Spirit within us stirring it up. Truly, apart from Him we can do nothing, including dream of good things (John 15:5). So if God planted a seed of good desire in our hearts, we can trust Him to bring the harvest He intended for that desire. His heart for us is always loving, good, and for our freedom and joy, so we can trust Him to finish the good work He started in us. But, as all seed and creation experiences, there is no fruit without first a death.

NOT SO SWEET SURRENDER

We experienced the peak of fall foliage in our region a few weeks ago. It was stunning. We almost thought we wouldn't have a dramatic transition this year. We had leaves clinging dressed in a rich dark green for weeks, refusing to give way to change. At last, though, our streets and hills glowed with coppers, every shade of mustard, amber, brick reds, and orange. My little family slept in one morning during the peak so we could enjoy bacon, eggs, and pancakes before heading out for a hike along a beloved local trail to see the Laurel Falls in Tennessee. As we rested on mini-summits along the way, and paused to take in the breathtaking views of the foothills, we thanked each other for being family to us. We were overcome by the goodness surrounding us in human, and hill, form.

But our hike was a wee bit longer than we planned. We got lost.

Why they bother to have trailhead signs with colors associated with trails, when they fail to mark trees with the color partway through the trail, is beyond me. Mark the trees, trail people. Especially when the way is forked.

We knew we were lost when we beached at a wide, raging river. There was no going any further, unless we wanted to die in the crossing. I think for a moment my grizzly bear husband considered it! He pointed to a trail on the other side of the raging river and said, "The trail is supposed to keep going over there."

I told him that was fine but the point remained that there was a raging river between the trail we were on and the trail that picked up over there. Our desired destination was likely not far along that continued trail on the other side, but there was no way we were going to make it that way, at least not for me and my daughter!

We ended up turning around, backtracking a mile or so, then got on another path (marked with the wrong color for the trail, mind you). Eventually, two hours later than we anticipated, we made it to our destination.

While it is perfectly reasonable for me to resist raging rivers in this life, and while it is my job as my daughter's Mama to protect her from dangers like this with my very life, this is actually the place Jesus calls us to join Him. Regularly.

Some call it surrender.

Jesus calls it death.

Either way, I tend to resist this place, too.

To surrender my desires to the desire of God for my life feels like death. Jesus says it feels like death because it is death. Not for death's sake, though. Death, so that new life can spring up from it! With Jesus nothing is ever dead except our sin and shame, and the sad fate of death itself. Jesus doesn't fear death because there is nothing to fear when you have the power to resurrect—to bring life from the dead. In His river of surrender there is death, but also a new life that rises to meet a path on the other side that leads to a glorious destination.

We believe this is true for our souls, and look forward to the resurrection of our bodies and a glorious day when we all discover what we are truly like. But, what if in the resurrection we find all the dreams that died are resurrected? When we surrender our dreams to take up Christ's plans for our lives, I wonder if our dreams somehow go to paradise and in their place new dreams resurrect that stretch out further and wider in goodness beyond what we could have ever imagined.

EXPECTING RESURRECTION

How we pray is shaped by what we are expecting. If I'm expecting bad things to happen to me or my family, my prayers are fear-drenched petitions for safety, for protection, and for evil to be kept far from us. But if I'm expecting God to open up doors of restoration, healing, and blessing, my prayers are full of thanks and trust as I ask God to give me wisdom. I see this plainly in my daughter's requests of us, too. When she is expecting us to take her to the doctor for a flu shot, she begs us to assure her it won't hurt too badly, that it will be quick, that we will hold her hand, and that we will go get ice cream afterward. She is expecting pain, so her focus is on comfort and how quickly she can get to it. But when we are headed to her beloved Dollywood, she is expecting joy! She imagines us riding rides and holding hands all through the park. She is expecting fun, so her focus is on getting there and staying there as long as possible.

When our dreams go unfulfilled, month after month and year after year, we begin to wonder if these dreams are not the dreams God is shaping for our lives here. We resist at first, maybe in denial, that these dreams will in fact die. We resist because of what we are expecting with that death. We scramble for comfort and clamor for assurance that we will get through this visit quickly and as pain-free as possible.

As we neared the end of our first year trying to conceive and realized we were entering into "infertility," I began expecting my dream of bearing children would die. I expected heartbreak along with insatiable longing and emptiness in our home. I soon saw no hope of legacy, no hope of a big family I had always wanted, no joy in passing down traditions, and no celebration of life continuing on from ours. It was bleak. It felt personal. I wrestled with deep doubts that God loved me, believing that He loved other women more than me because they were good and I was bad.

Then when we started infertility treatments, I expected to get pregnant. I expected my dream would resurrect into a new life, just through medical intervention. My heart was hopeful, light, and curious again to see how God would provide. Then as months passed with no development, I began expecting the worst again. As we prepared for my endometriosis surgery, I buoyed back and expected it to "cure" whatever our "problem" was, and to conceive the first month out. I remember being peaceful going into surgery, wishing I could have conceived without it but grateful that we seemed to be nearing the finish line of our struggle. Then when several months passed with no signs of life within, I began expecting God was punishing me, and would continue. I felt like I was being rejected for being uniquely unlovely and was disqualified from receiving His blessing.

We can only truly release our dreams in surrender when we expect Jesus to make all things new.

This way of living was not only miserable, it was based on poor theology.

In Jesus' economy, when a thing dies that is good, it falls to the earth, is buried, and then rises up to new life. It is just His way. I was living with a mindset saddled with shame and fear, believing that every death is final and pronounces a condemning judgment against me. This belief stands in direct opposition to the gospel! Jesus took all my condemning judgment in His own body when it was nailed to the cross. That fateful day, whatever was wrong with me went on wood with blood, then to a tomb, and died a final death. It was finished. All the worst outcomes and all the deaths ended there in a tomb. And when Jesus rose up three days later, in His mysterious way He made *all our dreams* come true.

We can only truly release our dreams in surrender, though, when we expect Jesus to make *all* things new. We can only bring our dreams to the altar of God's will, and let them die, when we expect Jesus to bring resurrection.

PRAYING FOR RESURRECTION

My talks with my daughter about life after death are enjoyable because we live with hope in resurrection. We talk about it, we look forward to it, we see evidence of it all around us in creation, and we pray with it in mind.

Just a few weeks ago we were getting ready in my bathroom when my daughter said completely out of the blue, "Mommy, I want a baby brother." To be exact, she wants twins. She actually asked over a year ago, and for a short while we were expecting twin boys through adoption, but they ended up being redirected to another family. That was a tough blow, too. It seemed like God opened the door and answered not only our prayers, but hers as well, then in the end He withheld them from us. We learned later details that gave us peace with the redirection, but I sometimes still wonder what that was all about.

I looked into my daughter's deep, dark-brown eyes that day, which shine just like mine, and saw her wide-open heart asking for what she desired. I love this about her. She understands there are things we say "no" to, but in her mind any dream of her heart is possible. I want her to stay this way. As her mother, I want to keep hearing the desires of her heart because they tell me about what she loves, what she thinks, what she enjoys and dreams about. Ultimately, I see her when I *hear* her heart, and she will discover someday that her openness will help her see herself and the God who made her.

We have a way of directing those desires and dreams, though, in our prayer for resurrection. With her request for a baby brother, we pass it on to Jesus (especially because even if I could conceive, I just cannot simply make a baby brother for her!). I want to teach my daughter what I am learning: to be dependent on Jesus for all things, and to pray and dream with Him from her heart. We teach her to ask, "Jesus, will You please give us a baby brother?" Then we look at each other, and together we remember out loud that Jesus resurrects and makes all things new. She then finishes her prayers this way: "Jesus, thank You for making all things new. You know best, and You will give us what is best for us."

No matter how much I want to have my way in this life, the gospel has seen to it that my old self with its own way, as well as sin and shame, are dead. The life I live now, I live in Christ, trusting His will for me is best for me. It is in His kindness and mercy that He gives me what is best for me and withholds what is not good for me (Psalm 84:11; 127:1). The enemy of God would love to stir this truth up in fear, tempting me to focus on all the suffering I will face in God's will, but this is not God's Spirit at work in me (Romans 8:15). God's sovereign power over my life helps me take comfort in peace that no matter what suffering I face, nothing will keep me, my family in Christ, or my dreams from resurrecting.

This doesn't mean I will always like His will for my life. I will not always bend my knees and submit my will to His willingly or cheerfully.

Death is still *death*. And I am still *human*.

I have the same mind of Christ (1 Corinthians 2:16) but sometimes I lack the perspective of God. I get glimpses of His way of seeing (Isaiah 55:8), but I don't know what He knows unless He reveals it to me. I don't see what He sees unless He opens my eyes. Often my anchor in these times when I teeter on the shore of my raging river is that I know His heart for me is good. I remember His resurrection of His own body, of Lazarus, and of my resurrection coming. I remember His opening of Sarai's womb and His own sealed tomb. I remember His faithfulness to Israel and to His Church. In a thousand ways I can recall His faithfulness to me over these forty-one years of living. I remember His faithfulness to so many who chose to trust Him when the future seemed uncertain (Hebrews 11). I remember that no matter which dreams may live, or which may die, He will be with me every step of the way (Deuteronomy 31:6).

No matter which dreams may live, or which may die, He will be with me every step of the way.

By His grace, I make the choice to trust God again.

For the joy of resurrection before me, I yield my dreams to Jesus who stands in the raging river.

I trust in the One who collects dreams when they die, carries them to paradise, and with resurrection power, makes all things new.

Natasha's Story

I know the rise and fall of hope for something long desired and the pain of loss when that dream dies. In my case it came before our journey with infertility. It was with my desire for marriage. I wish I could say that my desire for marriage was this beautiful and healthy longing. I knew marriage was a beautiful gift of God; but, somewhere along the way, I let getting married answer the question of whether I was valuable and worthy. I thought if a man approved of me, and married me, then I had finally "arrived." I was desperate to feel secure and loved, to overcome that gnawing fear that I didn't quite measure up as a woman. And I feared rejection above all.

Rejection came, though, in my late twenties. My fiancé called off our wedding just six weeks before the big day. I was devastated. The breakup felt like a confirmation of all that I feared was true about me: that I was fundamentally unworthy, unlovable, and unqualified for marriage. Even after I realized God actually saved me from a huge mistake, the insecurity from the rejection persisted. In my mid-thirties, my hurt had rooted and grown into bitterness over my unmarried state. To me, my singleness screamed out to the world that I was unworthy of love, fundamentally flawed, and not a real woman. I even believed God felt this way, too. To make matters worse, my younger sister had been married for nearly ten years, had three beautiful children, and wore my mother's stamp of approval.

When I turned thirty-four, maybe due to my biological clock pounding, I began to pursue marriage by putting myself "out there" primarily in the world of online dating. I also began to ask God to help me. Those ended up being two often divergent approaches, though. My pursuit of marriage was desperate and frenzied. I wanted to get married as soon as possible, and even made some very poor choices that left me struggling with more shame. God's approach, however, was slow and methodical. Too slow for me! In my hubris, at times, I actually accused Him of doing nothing to answer my prayer for the desire of my heart.

During this time I had several confrontations with God. The first was when He gently addressed some destructive choices I made in a prior relationship. He confronted my belief about my own unworthiness and helped me realize that I actually grieved Him by acting out of the flawed belief that I am not worthy. He reminded me that He was my Creator and the Authority on all things concerning me, and that He says I am worthy. I am fearfully and wonderfully made by Him, who knit me together in my mother's womb (Psalm 139:13,14). He challenged me with this thought: "If you don't start believing the truth that you are worthy, you are calling Me a liar." Oh, how convicting... and wonderfully hopeful at the same time!

God also confronted my self-prescribed remedy (a husband), and showed me that this was not the answer for my insecurity. My real problem was that I was comparing myself to my sister and was weighing my mom's approval of me as more important than what God said about me. My mother had her own hurts, and bitterness even, from wounds in her marriage. In her bitterness, she injured me. And in my bitterness, I injured myself further. But through my deep desire for marriage, God led me to confront these seemingly unrelated, yet totally related, idols in my heart. God was lovingly curing me at the source of my diseased thinking!

Still, I felt like I was too old and running out of time. Men wanted younger women and God was going too slow. His pace felt like a denial of my desire. As I felt my former dream of marriage and family slowly dying, I grew angry and bitter again. So I knew my dream of marriage needed to die. In a Job-like confrontation (I actually was studying in the book of Job), God brought me to the realization that He is God and I am not. Who was I to tell the Great Physician what the prescribed remedy was when I didn't even understand myself enough to diagnose my real problem? With that, I broke. My attitude toward Him and His healing work was utterly wrong. Everything He had given me was enough. *He* was my answer to wholeness and worthiness. *He* was and is enough for me. Later

God gave me a new dream for marriage—one that did not come with all the pressure for a man to affirm me and make me whole. By God's amazing grace, despite my years of bitterness and anger toward Him, He gave me the new desire of my heart and I met my husband.

UPROOT

What do you believe about your dreams? What do you believe about dreams that seem to die? How are these beliefs hindering your faith from growing, or your hope from being full yet?

PLANT

How could believing what God says change your current beliefs?

PART TWO

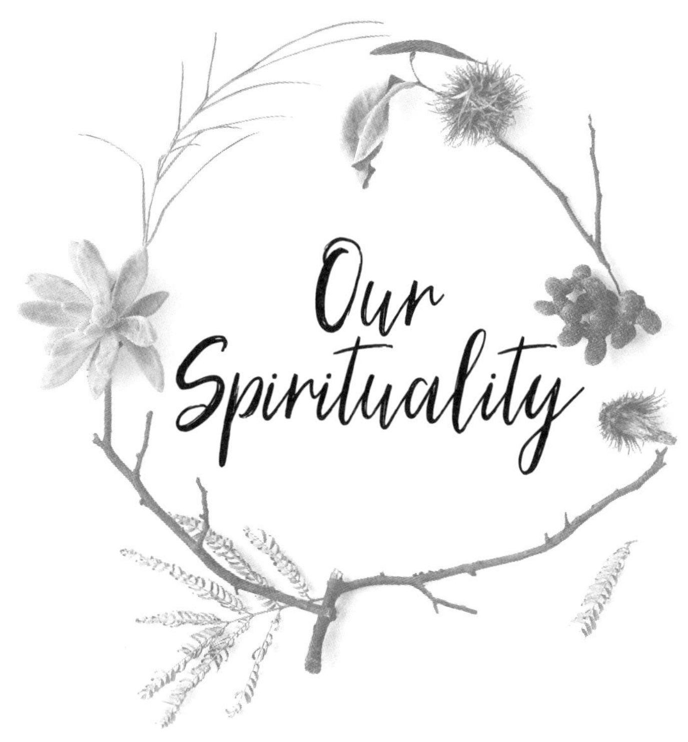

CHAPTER 7

A New Symbol of Life

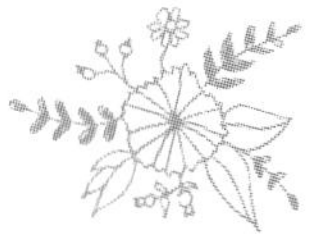

"Whoever desires to come after Me, let him deny himself, and take up his cross, and follow Me."

—Mark 8:34

We were in my car driving, my daughter and the most delightful teen girl on the planet. We were on our way home after church to get ready for a large gathering on our farm. The teen girl is the daughter of one of my dearest friends and babysits my daughter sometimes. She always astounds us with her tenderness and maturity even though she is only fifteen years old. There is hope for our children! I love moments shared with her and her younger sister. Both girls are growing under parents who shape their hearts to feel safe in love. A heart that feels safe in love is simply the most beautiful thing in the world to experience.

We were nearing the house when my daughter groaned from her car seat in the back, "I can't grab the shadow! Urgh! Mommy,

I'm trying to grab this shadow and I can't grab it!" The teen girl and I looked at each other in the rearview mirror and tried to hide our giggles. At the same time, though, I was struck by the depth of truth behind her exasperation. Being the nerd I am, I set out to explain to the beloved teen girl why my daughter's frustration was so meaningful. *That poor dear.* I need to go back and pay her extra. She was held hostage by a woman who loves words, and nerds out by discovering Scripture in everyday places.

I explained to her that in some way we are all grabbing for shadows. Grasping and groaning, we spend chunks of our precious lives trying to catch something that isn't actually there. All the while, it was merely pointing us to see the real thing.

THE WAY OF THE SHADOW

I'm not a science-y kind of person, having failed both organic chemistry and biology in my sophomore year of college. In the same semester. But I love learning from creation all I can about truth, goodness, wisdom, and the heart of God. So when I heard my daughter trying to grab at shadows, it intrigued me to consider the way of the shadow.

What a shadow tells us is that there is light. It is actually the undeniable proof of the presence of light. It is impossible to have a shadow without light. It also tells us there is a real thing. A shadow is undeniable proof of the presence of a real thing. A shadow, though, is neither the light nor the real thing. It is a darkness that hides and yet confirms that light and the real thing exist.

We may not notice the light or the real thing, though, even though we are very near to both. Sometimes we are just stuck looking in the direction of the shadow. The shadow steals all our attention with its distortion and mystery. We can follow shadows, even chase them, and grab at them. But we never, ever grab ahold of the shadow.

Just as there are shadows of everyday kinds all around us, the shadow is a shadow itself. There is a certain kind of shadow that points us to a Light and a real thing, but makes us stumble after it. And the tricky thing about this kind of shadow is that we can be trying to grab it without even knowing it.

SHADOWS WE TRY TO GRAB

In my twenties I prayed daily for a spouse. I had been engaged in college, but God intervened to call me out before I stepped into a relationship permanently that would have brought major regret. For both of us. After that, I became especially cautious about dating.

I began seeking God to understand better His love and plans for my life. I discovered how Jesus loved us as His bride, and paid all our debts just to gain our hand in marriage forever. It thrilled my heart to know He was making a Home ready for us with plans to host a wedding feast, the likes of which this world has never seen. My eyes opened and my focus shifted from the small story I was stuck in, longing for a husband, and realized it was all a shadow!

Marriage was important, blessed by God and to be valued, but it was still a shadow pointing us to the real thing—the wedding of Jesus and the Church soon coming. The light of God's Truth was illuminating the real thing for me that season, and I experienced new desires to care for His bride like a bridesmaid would, not chasing my own happiness for once. God's best plans for me would include a husband years later, but He continues to remind me that though this relationship is a gift, it is also a shadow. It will never be perfect because it is not the real thing, and it will never be the light, but it can help me see better how God's story is unfolding in mine.

You would think that lesson would help me recognize other shadows more easily, but no. As I chased food to comfort my anxiety, He revealed the shadow of food. It was a filling, a comfort, a kind of nourishment that is actually a shadow of the real thing found in God's Word. Slowly I began to choose the real thing over the shadow, and filled my soul with the finest bites in Scripture. Later as I chased jobs, titles, and status, He revealed the shadow of importance. I wanted to grab onto a purpose, a meaning, a secure identity, for which the world offers shadows of all kinds. The real thing, though, is found in being a child of God with a special contribution to the mission of building up His Kingdom. Slowly I began to choose the real thing, an identity in Christ where I have a purpose and gifts to build up others, no matter what I achieve in this world.

I thought I was becoming an expert at shadow spotting, but we all have our own kind of shadow blinders. When I longed to be a mother of children, I thought this was the real thing, too. "Be fruitful and multiply" was a command for God's children to build families, right? Spending money and energy in pursuit of childbearing felt right, good, even a command of God. And let me say this clearly: I do not believe it was wrong to do so. We are free to dream and pursue our dreams. When that dream becomes an obsession, though, and when not getting it devastates us so that we refuse to obey God's leading, then our dream has become an idol. This is not good. Not because it makes God small, because nothing we do can make Him small. Chasing idols is not good because they damage us, and God loves us too much to let us damage ourselves without drawing us back to Him.

During our season with infertility treatments, when I was on staff leading our women's ministry, we hosted a conference featuring leading Bible teachers and pastors including Nancy Leigh Demoss (now Wolgemuth), John Piper, and others. It was a lovely day, and I was trying to listen as I scurried around behind the scenes sorting the catered lunch and reviewing the schedule. I was grateful to have a job that kept my mind and heart occupied in the direction of truth those days. And on that day in particular. As I stacked box lunches, I heard Nancy speak truth that would alter the course of my life.

Nancy at the time was in her fifties and had never been married. She had faithfully pursued the will of God for her life, served Him with her whole heart, and that meant never marrying (at least at that point) and bearing children. Listening to her wisdom in my early twenties would have been off limits by me, because I would have been afraid of this being God's call for me too. But now I was intrigued by her joy, her peace, her delight in the midst of not getting what I thought were the twin joys for most women: marriage and children. I was gently rolling this paradox around in my mind when she said these words, and I'm going to paraphrase: "God does not grow His family through procreation, but through regeneration by faith in Christ."

I had an unstoppable seed of life within me that could regenerate new life in others through faith.

I stopped dead in my tracks. And in a hidden way, my shadow chasing stopped dead, too.

The truth spoken in those words nailed my flesh all over again to Christ's cross and set my soul free from chasing a shadow I had been trying to grab without realizing it. I was believing the shadow of pregnancy was the real thing. All the while, I already had the real thing. I had life growing inside of me because of the gospel of Jesus Christ. I had an unstoppable seed of life within me that could regenerate new life in others through faith. I had already shared the gospel with many in my lifetime, experiencing the beauty of new birth firsthand, so the truth was *I was already a mother.* I just didn't know it.

I kept that truth close to my heart for a few days before I sank fully into what it meant for my life. At home, on my living room floor in grief after getting news that yet another woman I knew was expecting a baby, I surrendered my life to the real thing. I stopped chasing the shadow of pregnancy. God in His grace opened my eyes and lifted my gaze to what the light of truth was pointing to: my ability to grow God's family by faith. In the quietest moments alone with God, through my tears of surrender, I believe He let me see my dining room table in Heaven. It stretched into the streets surrounded with children on all sides, laughing and sharing stories. Like a loving whisper over my shoulder I felt Him say, "You grow My family, and let Me grow yours."

Like a loving whisper over my shoulder I felt Him say, "You grow My family, and let Me grow yours."

Our prayer had been for years, "Lord, grow our family in quality and in quantity." He showed me He had seeded that prayer in my heart during my single years, because it was the desire of His own heart. Now, with my dreams surrendered to Him, He resurrected new dreams with that new vision. I didn't have to wait any longer to own my role as a mother. When I got up off the floor, like Deborah, *I rose as a mother* (Judges 5:7).

A NEW SYMBOL

If I could get back the money I have spent on pregnancy tests, even in the last few months, I could purchase a time-share on a coast. The cheap ones can leave you frustrated with vague results, so you go and buy the expensive good ones anyway. The anticipation of finding out if you are carrying life within is agonizing, whether you are hoping for the news to be positive or not. It's the longest couple of minutes of your life. But for those who are deeply longing to carry a child, we know what that well-known symbol of life is supposed to look like:

+

I've never seen one, for the record. I cannot imagine the feeling of actually seeing this pop up on one of those little white sticks. It must be the most exhilarating feeling for a couple who has been trying to conceive for so long. Perhaps the longer the struggle, the more overwhelming the joy.

But for those who never get the plus sign, or who lose it quickly, what is *our* hope? Does this little symbol really have the power to tell us whether we have life within us? If this is just a shadow of a real thing, what is the *real* thing?

I believe God gave me a new symbol of life. Well, just new to me, really. And I want to offer it to you today, too.

If pregnancy is a shadow of the expectant hope we can have when we have the gospel implanted in our souls, what then is the symbol of life indicating to the world that we are expecting? You may be shocked to see that it is nothing new, not really:

+

Did you catch that?

It's the cross.

The cross of Christ is a symbol of life for those whose sins and shame were washed away on it. The cross of Christ is a sure sign that you, darling daughter or son of God, have life within you, right now. No matter what a white stick has ever said, you are expecting life. You can expect Jesus to do good in and through you.

The real thing says so, and we can believe it and learn to let go of the shadows.

THE REAL THING

I had a vague understanding of the gospel before our infertility journey. Even though I had been reading God's Word for nearly two decades, participated in missions focused on evangelism, and even taught and served in ministry for years, my deep love for the gospel itself didn't grow until I experienced my own complete inability to bear life of my own. The real thing that gives me life and confirms I have life within me is due to the cross of Jesus Christ. The blood shed for me on Jesus' cross promises me I have the gospel seed within me that can revolutionize my world. I am no longer barren. Instead, I have the ability to bring change to my world through the unstoppable and reproducible life of Jesus. Now, I'm a revolutionary.

The enemy of God would love for us to believe we have nothing to offer, or no legacy to leave behind, if we do not bear children or do other amazing things with our lives. This is far from true, though, because the seed we bear is unstoppable. It can bear life in impossible situations. Gospel seed can break through the hardest blockages; it can reach beyond seas and government lockdowns. The seed of Christ in us triumphed over sin and shame. It triumphed over death. It transcends time and space and is fully able to transform our stories. I had been "with child" for decades and didn't know it. There is potential for us to bear fruit in our lives that cannot be measured. We can literally parent thousands of children by faith, while even one child is meaningful.

One day, overwhelmed by self-pity, I felt God nudge my spirit, reminding me of what Jesus and His disciples did on the earth with their lives. I thought, "Yeah, that was them but this is me." I heard Him speak gently but directly to my heart: "The same God who spoke to the apostle Paul and C. S. Lewis speaks to you, Heather." God was not and is not a respecter of persons. I was not the only exception to His promise to use ordinary women and men to build His family. But I had a choice. I could accept that I was pregnant with the gospel and could bear life, or I could deny it. I could be a conduit of grace, or shut down in self-pity and shame.

Thankfully, friends, God woke me up. So today, I'm expecting. And you can be too. Maybe, though, you need to see a new symbol of life. I hope you see it soon, because:

We are the disciples.

We are the life-bearers.

We are the mothers and fathers.

We are no longer barren. Now, we can be revolutionaries.

May we take up our cross, embrace our symbol of life, and live like pregnant women expecting Jesus to move in and through us.

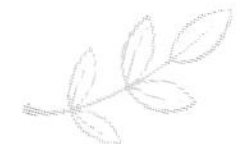

Lydia's Story

When I married, I brought with me hopes that I could finally become a parent in my thirties. I had a desire for motherhood that laid fertile inside my soul for years. So when five years into marriage, we learned we would not have children, my world suddenly looked unrecognizable, my future a dark shadow. I wrote privately, "This is the loss of hopes and dreams for the last thirty years or so... I feel like there's a hole in my heart, this ache that recurs... I stand in His strength because it's the only strength I have. I will repeat, until I believe it deep in my soul, that God knows the best plan for my life."

And that's what I did through those next months, praying repeatedly, proclaiming a trust that I did not feel.

Unbroken years of emptiness stretched ahead of me, and I didn't know what to look forward to, except to somehow keep serving Jesus and loving my husband. I asked God, "Why me? What could You possibly have for me that's better than motherhood?" I journaled later, "It's been a year! I'd like to not cry so easily… I want to move on. But just saying it doesn't make it so."

Somehow, God took my feeble efforts at trust and began bringing a new hope to my life. Slowly, like a new plant unfurling from the soil, I gained a new confidence from outside myself as I took new risks and began building community around me. My baby steps of faith bore fruit. God gave me a vision of what life could be—and it was like light breaking into a darkened room. I felt hope again, hope for a purpose and joy that did not depend on my circumstances. And even now, years later, that hope does not disappoint. God is faithful.

UPROOT

What beliefs do you hold for the roles you play, or don't play, today (wife, mom, grandmother, boss, friend, rocket scientist, and so on) that are holding you back from seeing a bigger role God is offering you?

PLANT

How could believing these roles are shadows change the way you see your life?

CHAPTER 8

Every Mama Has Her Limits

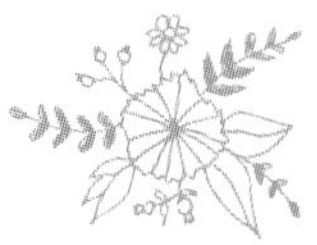

"Without Me you can do nothing."

—John 15:5

I recently saw a post online by a popular speaker, author, and social media influencer speaking to a roomful of women selling products under a multi-million-dollar brand. One word was displayed above her head to capture the heart of her message:

Limitless.

I knew what she meant, I think. After reading other posts, I filled in the gaps with more context and soon I realized we see limits differently.

To her, limits hold you back. Limits block you from getting what you want. Limits are artificial, made up in our minds due to self-limiting thoughts that keep us from becoming all we are meant to be. Limits were to be broken through, dismissed, looked past because on the other side of every limit is the life we want.

And her point was we can all have the life we want.

Here is what we agree on, because I like to build on what we share with others as often as possible! There are times when we are being held back by self-limiting thoughts that are based on lies. Lies work in our minds to cripple us from being able to walk straight and plant our feet firmly on the ground laid before us. It is wise to filter our thoughts regularly so we extract the self-limiting lies and make decisions based on what God says about us.

There are also limits that others may put on us that are not from God. Recently I came to terms with a painful realization that even people I love may not support me in following God's path for me. Whether it comes in the form of rejection, or well-intentioned but poor advice, or even an overt attempt to derail us, if we base our decisions on the limiting opinions of others, we may not fulfill God's purposes in our lives. Maybe you recognize this behavior in a relative or friend, or maybe a teacher or boss who is telling you what to be when you grow up. Sometimes people try to lovingly warn us of choices that lead to wasteful lives, and we need that kind of tough love. But sometimes people put limits on us that are just not from God. Whatever is not of God, you are free to release.

There are times when we are being held back by self-limiting thoughts that are based on lies.

Sometimes we release a belief, and in some cases we may need to release a person with forgiveness and grace (not your spouse). It won't be easy. In fact, we may have to fight with the hounds of Hell bent on our oppression. Every time I released ungodly self-limiting beliefs or the limits put on me by other people, I experienced a painful and confusing cut that tempted me to doubt God. On the other side of these cuts, though, I would eventually discover joy in freedom to follow Jesus as closely as possible. And freedom like this is indescribably wonderful.

LIMITS THAT FREE US

When Jonathan and I got married, we had both lived a lot of life and learned from many wise couples what not to do if we wanted to build a healthy marriage. For example, we were both sharp witted, and sarcasm was like a second language for us. But coming into courtship we kept our communications clear, direct, sincere, and open, and didn't bring sarcasm into our relationship.

Until one day.

One Saturday while we were driving we talked about how our communication felt so "clean"—we just said what we meant with openness and vulnerability without couching it in passive or hostile terms. We shared how sarcasm was a part of our speech before, though, and so for a few moments we tried it in the car.

It was awful. It felt like another person stepped into Jonathan's body, and a different woman in mine, and they didn't like each other very much.

We both decided right then and there that we were adopting a zero-tolerance policy on sarcasm for our relationship. Joking and teasing were acceptable, within limits (no name calling that belittled, or making fun of body parts ever). But sarcasm would need to go. In fact, we decided that if we found ourselves in sarcasm, the one at the receiving end had the right to go open the front door and call the other to come spit it out. Zero tolerance. A limit. And it has produced more joy and health in our communications than any other limit on our speech!

Another limit we placed on ourselves was with regard to sharing spaces with the opposite sex. We committed to never eat at a restaurant alone with someone of the opposite sex, never ride in a car alone, never be in a room alone without it having a window or an open door, and never "hang out" alone as friends with someone of the opposite sex. Now, there have been times when Jonathan has had appointments with elderly widows at their homes because driving is difficult for them, so obviously we use wisdom and have leniency in matters that make sense, but you get the idea. The limits we place on ourselves are not to keep us from having fun, hinder our enjoyment of freedom, or hold us back from becoming who we are made to be—quite the opposite! Like guardrails on a highway, these limits protect what we love most: each other. The trust we build because of the boundaries in place only enhance our fun and our enjoyment of freedom.

These limits are fairly easy to see as reasonable and helpful, even undeniably wise. But there are limits that are harder to recognize, that get blurry to discern because they can appear to be harsh and cruel at times. We all benefit from limits, though, of all kinds. We are not made to be limitless; the Bible tells us so. We are made to be so limited, in fact, that we can do nothing of eternal meaning apart from God's grace. It is in discovering these limits, embracing them without shame, and resting in God to be the only One who is limitless, that I believe we come to taste real freedom.

SARAI'S LIMITS

If ever an adoption plan failed to pan out, Abram and Sarai's story is the one. In fact, trying to pursue an adoption plan seemed to only inflame Sarai's pain of infertility grief as well as Hagar's struggles. Hagar's "despising" of Sarai is unclear, but regardless of what she was doing, Sarai was constantly reminded that other women could do something she couldn't do. She couldn't escape her inability to have a child, and now couldn't escape an angry birthmother and an incredibly hostile home dynamic. When women have babies around women who cannot have babies, things just aren't simple. It is a mysterious grace that adoption is ever possible for families when emotions run so deep.

In reading Sarai's story, it is easy to judge her for being impulsive, focused on having a child, and then drawing a harsh line with Hagar. But even Sarai had her limits. The infertility grief now coupled with strife and marital tension were too much for her to bear, and I imagine the woman was desperate for some space from it all. But whatever regret Sarai carried over her broken relationship with Hagar, and over her troubles with Abram, God did *not* reject her. We just need to turn the page to see His heart for her, too.

> Then God said to Abraham, "As for Sarai your wife, you shall not call her name Sarai, but Sarah shall be her name. And I will bless her and also give you a son by her; then I will bless her, and she shall be a mother of nations; kings of peoples shall be from her." (Genesis 17:15,16)

Not only was God going to give her the desires of her heart, a child, God was going to put an end to the memory of her past self. Her prior desperate efforts, her broken relationships, her harsh dealings were all washed away. She was a new woman in God's eyes, but God wanted her to see herself as new too, and gave her a new name. God changed her name from Sarai, meaning "she who strives," to Sarah, meaning "lady, princess, princess of the multitude."[7] Some commentaries suggest both names contained the meaning of "princess" but the latter added the implication of "multitudes." The point is God was declaring Sarah as part of the covenant He was making to build His kingdom. Abram would now be Abraham, a "father of many nations" (Genesis 17:5), and Sarah would be a "mother of nations."

Can you imagine this woman's heart? I just sit here thinking about her and tears are spilling out of my eyes. I mean, this woman has *been through it.* She feels misunderstood, judged, brokenhearted, longing, weak and desperate, lacking belief, distant from God, guilty, ashamed, loaded down with grief, confusion, and regret. Then she wakes up the next day and learns she is now "God's lady, a princess." But it gets better. Soon it would not just be Abraham, or Hagar, to whom God speaks, but it becomes Sarah's turn to encounter this God of the universe for herself.

> Then they said to him, "Where is Sarah your wife?" So he said, "Here, in the tent."
>
> And He said, "I will certainly return to you according to the time of life, and behold, Sarah your wife shall have a son."
>
> (Sarah was listening in the tent door which was behind him.) Now Abraham and Sarah were old, well advanced in age; and Sarah had passed the age of childbearing. Therefore Sarah laughed within herself, saying, "After I have grown old, shall I have pleasure, my lord being old also?"
>
> And the LORD said to Abraham, "Why did Sarah laugh, saying, 'Shall I surely bear a child, since I am old?' Is anything too hard for the LORD? At the appointed time I will return to you, according to the time of life, and Sarah shall have a son."
>
> But Sarah denied it, saying, "I did not laugh," for she was afraid. And He said, "No, but you did laugh!" (Genesis 18:9–15)

Let me just say I am in such good company with Sarah. I mean, she finally gets her shining moment with God and what does she do? She gets scared and lies. All I would add to the scene is quite possibly peeing my pants. But still, it was a life-altering encounter with her Creator all the same. As I close Sarah's story here, I'm left with this question by God to Sarah, and to all of us: *Is anything too hard for the Lord?* With God there is forgiveness, restoration, even legacy from barrenness. If it is possible for Sarai now Sarah, it is possible for us. No barrenness, no brokenness, no disaster is too hard for the Lord to redeem.

REACHING MY LIMITS

Reflecting on the moments that brought me to my limits, as they pertain to motherhood, has set off triggers of confusion, regret, and grief over the last couple of years. Only in the last several months have I been able to find hope in these spaces.

When we first brought our daughter home, we hoped to have some form of open relationship with our daughter's birthparents, as long as it was healthy for our family. I don't say "open adoption" for several reasons. First of all, in Tennessee there is no such thing. Every adoption is closed; any relationship you wish to have with people is voluntary. So, for that reason I refer to what we hoped to have as an "open *relationship*" that later became a "closed relationship." Also, a relationship is a living thing, so it can change and can go from open to closed, and even back to open again. This freedom from finality has been of great encouragement to me lately, remembering that Jesus can resurrect what feels dead.

As far as an open relationship in adoption goes, like in everything in life, expectations are everything. We expected, based on prior conversations, to set up one or two visits the first year with a birthparent. What we didn't expect was someone with the agency agreeing to terms that were not our terms. That person is no longer employed there, and apologized, but it was yet one more decision made for our family that we had to choose to embrace with surrender. There was no way we were going to allow for our witness of the love of Christ to seem unreliable when others were learning about God through our stories. So while we had no legal responsibility to comply with *any* visitation arrangement, we ended up meeting every two weeks for months. Thereafter, the visits would slowly be reduced to monthly, then bi-monthly, and so forth, like a weaning process.

There is a reason our adoption agency later said that this is never what they recommend to people. It was a heartbreaking experience for all of us.

I felt like at any moment I could "lose our daughter" because of a well-crafted accusation.

Each time we traveled for these visits, I'd have to stop before arriving because I was sick to my stomach. I'd grow increasingly anxious as the day neared, then would take a few days (or two weeks) to settle back down from the emotional jarring. During the visits Jonathan and I prayed continually, and would experience the peace of God sustaining us, but we noticed with each visit that our meetings together were not aiding healing. Despite our desire to have loving relationships with everyone involved, it became clear after the first month that our dynamic was going to be more challenging than any of us imagined.

By the second month relationships began deteriorating, boundaries were continually being crossed, and nothing we tried helped to facilitate peace and good will. By the third month words and behaviors became increasingly hostile toward us, me especially; and by the fourth month we felt endangered at times. When we attempted to establish boundaries for our physical and emotional health, we were instead met with more hostility. We were advised that our situation was extremely rare, just 1 percent of what our regional office experienced, and that it was not likely to ever improve for various reasons beyond our control.

During that season, I began experiencing panic attacks, and struggled against recurring fears that led me into a mild depression. Jonathan kept my cell phone when we were together and I kept it silent when I was home alone because the sound of text messages triggered anxiety. I felt like at any moment I could "lose our daughter" because of a well-crafted accusation, even though we were legally safe. In addition to fear of something happening to our family, or of losing our daughter, I felt enormous guilt for having our daughter and shame for not being able to help others heal. I had shared the love of Christ in words and action, and yet felt like I failed as a Christian witness, largely because this is one of the comments slung at me.

We wanted a door open for healing, peace, and emotional health so we could parent our daughter wholeheartedly, but it was not working for any of us. We didn't want to close the relationships, just the door to the harassment and cruel words being lodged against us, privately and later publicly. We live in a culture that rightfully honors parents who choose adoption for their child. It is a high form of love to give a child a life you feel is better than the one you can offer. I am forever humbled and grateful for this indescribable gift of parenting my daughter, and it's that gratitude that made it hard to put boundaries up to protect our family from harm. If I ended the connection, I worried I would confirm what was being said about me: I was a cruel woman, unfeeling and selfish, a disgrace to the Christian faith and a hypocrite.

We had very little advocacy available to help us at the time and pressure continued to mount around our relationship. Also, I had not yet resigned from my ministry position at our church, so I continued to oversee women's groups and events while my husband was taking over a large family business. Not to mention, we were adjusting as first-time parents of a newborn! Infertility grief was stirring up with a vengeance too, as I was continually reminded that my daughter didn't come from my womb. I felt cornered by verbal attacks, misunderstandings, grief, insecurity, dark emotions, confusion, and prayed for God to do a miracle.

Then God did. One of so many in our story.

God intervened on our behalf one fateful and hot Monday in July 2014 when we received an unexpected (and shocking) communication asking for no more meetings, no more letters, no more communications. They wanted to move on, to forget the past, and apologized for making our lives miserable. It was a bittersweet message. We wanted to build healthy relationships, but we felt God's hand providing an open door to healing for all of us, through the closing of that door of connection. We quickly acknowledged these wishes and confirmed that we would comply. The agency still required that letters be sent monthly for the first year to the office, so we would continue that for the agency, but otherwise we were done.

Thereafter I blocked contact information so I could physically close the door to that channel of heartache. I felt free, finally. In fact, I went outside with my daughter, carrying her against my chest, out into the sunlight and into our field where I began to weep over her. I wept for her biological ties that were cut that hour, and for the relief that we could bond together in a peace we had not yet fully known. I took a picture of us with my phone, of those tears in that light, because though I couldn't share the meaning behind those tears with anyone but my husband, I knew it was a holy moment. This mama had her limits, and I had witnessed God meet me at mine.

Our little girl's name is the blending of two words that together mean dark-haired beauty free from oppression (to honor her privacy, we choose not to print it). In that moment outside, I got a glimpse as to why God gave her this name. He had plans to cut her from ties that bind, in so many ways. And already, through her life, God was releasing me from some oppression, too.

We hoped that was the end of the heartache in those relational dynamics, at least until our daughter was grown enough to reasonably voice her own desires. We had been warned, though, that our struggles would likely never end. We had no idea what that would mean, but found out less than a year later when we started seeing boundaries crossed again. Communications began coming through in channels that were off limits, including to our places of work and our websites. We tried to appease the people involved, assure them we were all healthy, but it wasn't enough. We were accused of terrible things, and the narrative of our journey was being twisted. With every decision to move on and enjoy our family, I felt enormous guilt that I didn't know how to resolve. In my mind, Jesus has given me so many chances, how could I not do the same for others?

But in this case, and what counseling helped me accept much later, there was nothing more we could have done. We can never give or do enough to help others change. Only Jesus can be enough for us.

After seeking counsel from adoption specialists, counselors, lawyers and law enforcement, we were advised to get our concealed carry permits. I didn't want to hear or believe it, but it confirmed why I was feeling so afraid. Jonathan was strong for our family, and was prepared to draw hard lines to protect us from harm of all kinds, but I struggled to draw the line. At one point I went off most social media, stopped blogging, and then finally resigned from my position in ministry. I entered what I call now "the basement season" that lasted two years. I stopped using my real name online and began to seek counseling for infertility grief and post-adoptive trauma. I needed healing and a better understanding of how to own my limits.

My inability to sustain these open relationships was not the only experience that brought me to confront my "limits" during this season. Around this time, a teen girl I had mentored for many years was placed in a nearby group home. We were told she had no more family willing to house her, so I began visiting her on weekends, as she earned the time. Jonathan and I had been praying for her and eventually felt God was calling us into fostering, at least to provide a home for her until she could launch into college on more stable footing. We talked with social workers, counselors, and doctors, went through months of training and continued visits, and readied our house to bring her home.

I felt like the dreams that I had were crushed by God's will for me to suffer in serving others.

We did, and for months I took a teenager and toddler to playdates, doctor visits, court and social worker meetings, work shifts, school, parks, and grocery stores. I listened to very different aged females process their worlds, often in my car or kitchen. Some moments were so precious I imagine they are tucked into God's pocket for safekeeping, far from the threat of other moments that left me raw with exhaustion. It took months before I realized my physical health was steadily declining. Each month held new doctor appointments, more testing, and new medication to bring relief to my constant back pain, circulation issues, chest pain, abdominal spasms, and sleeplessness. It never dawned on me that unresolved guilt, fear, and stress were killing me, one week at a time.

Finally in the summer of 2016, Jonathan and I had a work trip that took us away for one week. Our petition to take our teen with us for a wonderful international experience was denied, so we arranged childcare with family. I could do only a fraction of our planned excursions because of pain and illness, and used my time stuck in bed alone to pray and read Scripture. I stayed connected to our kids, who seemed to be doing well, but my spirit was heavy with all kinds of mysterious burdens. On our way home, I felt even more poorly than my new normal and happened to check my calendar. There was a chance I could be pregnant, and time seemed to stand still as I wondered if this was what all the struggle was about, even the new battle with physical illness. I daydreamed that maybe this was the reward God had for us in the midst of all our challenges! I was cautiously hopeful, running my mind slowly over the dream of bearing children. Later that night, not only did I learn that I was not pregnant, but we got the call that we were actually expecting a new niece. As joyful as the news was, the timing of it felt like a cruel kick when we were already down.

As I turned to sleep that night, I struggled against a desire to not return home to my life. I felt like I was constantly failing someone and that nothing I did mattered or was enough. I felt like the dreams that I had were crushed by God's will for me to suffer in serving others despite how I was treated. I reasoned that if this was my cross, I wanted out. I wanted to go Home because I was a terrible cross-bearer and no one was being helped by me. The next day in the Atlanta airport I stood at a crossroads with Jesus. I was desperate for hope that this was *not* my new normal: handicapped physically and emotionally. Like many good crossroads, mine ended up in a public restroom. While awaiting our flight I hid crying in a tiny silver-walled stall with my Bible, and the tears wouldn't stop. (There's no telling what other women were thinking, but with only my feet showing and muffled sobs heard, I just didn't care anymore!) As I gushed out my anger and disappointment, I turned to a verse that brought hope I forgot was even possible:

> Is it not yet a very little while till Lebanon shall be turned into a fruitful field, and the fruitful field be esteemed as a forest? (Isaiah 29:17)

I didn't know what that meant for me, if anything at all, but even the remote hope of being "turned into a fruitful field" buoyed my soul up and out of my deep sorrow. I longed to bear fruit, and was believing a lie that there was no fruit in me, or that none could ever come from my life.

We returned home, and my heart clung to the hope of fruit. Things seemed to be fine, and the children seemed chatty and happy to see us. I swallowed the stirring burdens and blamed the jet lag as I clung to my hair-thin new hope.

Later that night, though, my thin hope bubble burst with news I never expected. Sparing the details, we discovered things that changed everything about our fostering dynamic. Suffice it to say, we didn't sleep at all that night. I pored through Scripture crying, overwhelmed with confusion, fear, anger, and grief. We knew we could not continue as we were, but my fear of being "un-Christ-like" paralyzed me from confronting evil and demanding respect for our limits. I found passages that I once read through a lens that made me feel guilty for owning my limits, but as I read them this time they illuminated in new ways. In their context, I began to see Jesus with dignity, giving dignity to others. I saw Jesus respect people's limits, never bullying or pressuring them to do what they didn't want to do. I saw Jesus allow for relationships to separate, and for ministry to still be fruitful. I saw reconciliation happen in the context of mutual repentance, but not be forced when someone was unwilling to own their part in it.

By the time the sun rose, I felt peace finally in being weak, limited, unable to save or serve people beyond God's grace. I felt free to have my own dignity and my own needs and to stop apologizing for them. I believed finally that I had a duty to protect what was important to me, including my heart, my health, my husband, my daughter, and my home. God gave us wisdom to call in our social worker to be present as we confronted the situation we were in, and gave us peace in offering one last chance to our teen before moving on with separation.

I had no idea how this was going to go, but we knew enough to expect a struggle. It only took a few minutes before we all knew the situation was beyond reconciliation, as far as the teen was concerned. I never even got a word in. The only words I did share were privately with the social worker when we started to sense some pushback along the lines of faith. Deep down I knew the battle was going to be along these lines, and thankfully God had prepared me for this in the night.

When the pushback came, I pulled forward to the edge of my seat to make sure both feet were planted squarely on the floor. Jonathan looked over at me and later said that it was at that moment when everything changed for us. I looked our social worker straight in the eye, and I think my soul was looking every person in the eye who ever tried to make me believe I was a failure because I had limits. I said, "I am not God. I am a woman, and I have limits. And today, I am done feeling sorry about this. This is not the first time I have been made to feel responsible for another person's choices and their well-being, and I'm done. I am not the Savior. In fact, I need Him myself. I have to believe that if I set even someone I love out on the curb, God can raise the ruins—but I know today, I cannot."

Jonathan said later that he knew something had shifted in me. He was right. It was a necessary moment, when something dropped off of me like a dozen backpacks I had been carrying in desert heat. The words rung in the air, and I was briefly tempted to feel cruel for them, when the social worker looked at me and said, "Well… that is truth."

Hours after the conversation began, the teen girl was escorted out with the social worker. The only words I said to her, through my tears, as she went out the door were, "It didn't have to be this way." It didn't for her, but it did for me. The social worker said a few last things to me before she left: "Heather, you are free. You have done nothing wrong here. You need to thank God, go play worship music, and praise Him for what He has done here today."

Failing to be "perfect" for another person is never fatal when we follow the One who raises ruins.

I learned every mama has her limits. And this is a good thing.

This is the gospel.

This new posture of freedom was critical when we decided to move forward seeking legal protection a year later responding to more harassment from a birthparent. It was no longer something I needed to wrestle with guilt and shame over, because I now trusted that God was able to bring life from the dead. Killing myself to keep something alive was not my responsibility. Since that day we have been in courtrooms owning our limits and trusting God. I have heard these words from a judge, "Mrs. Yates, tell us your story." I have grieved, and at the same time have continued to hold hope for restoration in the future.

But I'm no longer letting the enemy of God shame me for having limits.

We are given limits not only for physically parenting children, but this is true for our spiritual parenting as well. We just cannot save people. It nearly killed me trying to be God, to be everything for everyone. God created me to have limits and I was trying to live limitless believing this is what a "good Christian" was meant to be—but this was not true, and it was not the gospel. It was my pride. Jesus ripped this belief off of me, along with the heavy yoke of playing God, and began teaching me to carry His easy yoke instead (Matthew 11:30).

Discipleship is the process of spiritually maturing to become like Christ. Just as we grow up physically and achieve progress milestones, so too we grow spiritually. After putting our trust in Christ for salvation, we become new people. We are born new, into a spiritual family as adopted children of God. As such, we are mere infants, and can do nothing but receive "spiritual milk" and nurturing from God and spiritual mothers and fathers in His body, the Church. The intention is for us to grow up so we can learn to eat heartier meals of the Word, stand for ourselves on what God says about us, and begin learning how to walk in faith. We stumble, we fall, we get back into step with Jesus and keep learning a new life of following Him, responding to His love, and making choices from a new place of love. Growing mature is growing in our understanding of who we are and why we are here. There are many experiences along the way as we grow into spiritual mothers and fathers, and just like in adulthood, we get to own the choices we make.

But never ever does Jesus make us responsible for others' choices.

We are never empowered to be the Savior, only to point to Him. We are never inserted into another's life to be their Holy Spirit, only to pray they listen to Him. We are never equipped to meet all the needs of all the people, only to rise to the occasion as the Body of Christ as God guides.

Failing to be "perfect" for another person is never fatal when we follow the One who raises ruins. We need a Savior, too, and ultimately this is the best kind of discipleship experience we can offer our spiritual children. As I raise my daughter, I embrace my mistakes and own them in front of her. I acknowledge my sins, I confess them and repent or change course, and together we practice forgiveness and reconciliation. My hope is that she will grow up understanding her limits are nothing to hide, to ignore or be ashamed of, that they actually offer her access to the wide and deep love of God she needs. Her limits will protect her from sharing and living in a false gospel, where she is the hero of the story.

In true discipleship, there is one Hero. And this ain't you, Mama.

Jesus is the Hero for all of us, and He has no limits. What is impossible for us is possible with God (Luke 18:27). But as for the rest of us, the gospel bids us to own our limits, and find peace and freedom in Christ (Matthew 11:29).

I CANNOT CRY FOR YOU

One afternoon I saw a story on Facebook of a woman who died with young children. I didn't even know her but for several hours I cried, imagining the children and husband as if it could be my own family. By the time my husband came home, I was emotionally spent and had nothing left for my family that evening. It seemed ridiculous later, but at the time I grieved like she was my dearest friend, and this was a wake-up call for me. If I was going to move through my own grief well, and spend my best emotional energy on my family, I would have to choose who I cried over. I knew then that I needed limits on what I read, what stories I hear, and how I engage with sorrow in our world. Jesus came to save the world, but I came to be saved by Him and to point others to Him. If I was going to live my meaningful life well, I would need limits on who received my love and deepest compassion.

I also chose limits on my joy and celebration for others. For years, baby showers, social media baby bump journals, and Mother's Day church services were things I just needed to stay away from. Initially, I would try to be the happy woman wanting to celebrate others' joys, but the sadness would weigh me down so heavily I was exhausted and heartbroken for the remainder of the day, or days. It was not fair to my family to show up for others in a way that honestly didn't matter all that much to them, at the expense of being fully present and wholehearted with my husband. It was also not fair to my soul to drag it along to places where songs would be sung to my grieving heart.

The barren soul is never satisfied, because we are made to bear life. You *are made to bear life.*

There can yet be a time for celebration and joy in the future. For example, last spring a friend of mine, also with an infertility story, and I hosted a baby shower for another friend. We acknowledged to each other several times in the planning that this was ironic, even holy, that God would give us a lightness of step in an event that in the past knocked our knees out from under us. But I'll be honest, there are still times when a baby announcement, baby bump photo, or baby shower invitation stings. *The barren womb is never satisfied.* In a similar way, there are times when I fall for the old lie that I have nothing to offer. Or, I feel like I'm entering a spiritual menopause, growing irrelevant to my world. Maybe it's that the barren soul is never satisfied, because we are made to bear life.

You are made to bear life. You are made to build God's Kingdom alongside His people. But we remember that every mama also has her limits. We just cannot make life happen on our own. God wants to build His Kingdom through us, but with His strength, His agenda, and His power. He wants to raise the ruins and rebuild what has been torn down, but we cannot rebuild all the ruins ourselves.

> Unless the LORD builds the house, those who build it labor in vain. (Psalm 127:1, ESV)

Every mama has her limits, but every mama has her ruins to rebuild with God, too. What ruins are yours to rebuild with God? Maybe it's time to dream bigger...

Natasha's Story

I pushed my mama's limits. I was in my thirties with a law degree and a chip on my shoulder, because I was still single with no prospects. A few years earlier, at age twenty-nine, I was dumped a mere six weeks before my wedding and left with what seemed to confirm my greatest fear—that I really was not worthy or beautiful enough to be married. It hurt me to my core. I suffered crippling insecurity and bitterness toward men due to this rejection. But God led me to consider why this rejection had affected me so deeply, even using my screaming biological clock to motivate me to understand what was really going on in my heart.

God showed me that the root of my fear and insecurity was not about rejection by a man but by a woman: my mother. I always felt that I lacked her affirmation and approval as a woman, that she approved of and proudly associated with my sister, but not me. My younger sister had done it all the "right way" at the "right time" (married at twenty-four, first child at twenty-seven). The message I received was my sister was the standard and, compared to her, I was lacking.

The problem is, instead of letting God give me the affirmation I needed, I kept trying to get the approval from my mom. I believed two things at once: 1) I needed her approval so I would feel worthy of getting married and could attract a husband; and 2) I could win her approval once I was married. Wait. Which comes first? Yeah, it was illogical. And all about the approval of my mom!

And the illogical behavior continued. I would argue with her in an effort to get her to affirm me. I was trying to get her to understand why I needed her affirmation by making my case for why it's her fault I was insecure and, thus, unmarried. Predictably, that backfired. For her, all I was doing was dragging up her past and perceived failures, so she would defend herself.

I hit her limit one afternoon in May 2013. Once again we argued and I, again, attempted to make my case for why it was her fault I was still unmarried. She became so upset that she finally yelled at me, "Well, why don't you just kill yourself then?!" Whoa. While it was cruel, God gave me the grace to realize, first of all, that she didn't mean it; and second and more importantly, that my mom does not define my worthiness or set the standard for my ultimate approval. God does. My mom is a limited, finite, imperfect human being, and defining my worthiness is beyond her limits. I needed to let her off the hook. And I did right then, by God's grace. Fortunately, we forgave each other, and I stopped limiting God's ability to heal and affirm me. *He* affirmed me. I was worthy and beautiful.

UPROOT

How has believing you are, or have to be, "limitless" impacted you and your family negatively?

PLANT

How could embracing the truth that every mama (and person) has her limits shape your life today?

CHAPTER 9

Free to Dream Bigger

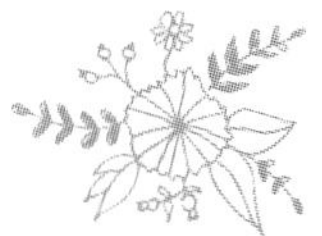

"And whatever you ask in My name, that I will do, that the Father may be glorified in the Son."

—JOHN 14:13

When I was twenty-seven years old and single, I was working in a law firm in Tallahassee, Florida, and was smack in the middle of a very challenging season in my journey. God had begun to peel back layers of hurt from my adolescence, and I felt like I was going backwards versus getting better. (I share this more in my first book, *All the Wild Pearls*, if you are interested.) Many nights I felt raw from the breaking He was doing to realign my heart with His Word. It was during one of those dark nights of the soul that I sensed Him whisper to my spirit calling me, "Little Flower." It was an odd moment, to say the least. I don't typically "hear God" in an audible voice, but I was crying out for comfort after the loss of my beloved grandmother, and was clinging to God for hope of any good in life ahead. I heard that name spoken over my heart and received it as best I could: "Little Flower." It felt so lovely, soft, and delicate. So I immediately rejected it. It didn't seem to fit me at all! Not the *me* I saw in me. But I sensed Him persist with me, and He showed me that my God-given name was Heather DeJesus for a reason. Translated, it meant "Little flower of/from the Lord."

I fell to my knees in that little apartment living room at the realization that God had made me to be lovely. The love of God flooded into my soul with such warm force that night, my sorrow gave way into joy as I began to dream again of all that was possible with Him. I felt lovely because I felt loved. While at the time I didn't understand what the significance of my name meant for my life, as it has played out God has entrusted me to speak to girls and adult women all over the world about His love. When I felt my most desperate for hope, like Sarai, God gave me hope through a new view of my name.

You'd think that with a name like "Little Flower," a writing and speaking ministry based on a succulent plant (*a mother of thousands*), and a home on a hay farm, I may be good at tending gardens. Funny fact: I kill plants like I get paid for it. No, really. I'm the worst. But I think this is the way of God, again. I think God chose to call a woman horrible with plants to tend women's hearts because I know this is not *my* work. Whatever good tending I get to do in others is *His* work through me. This recurring theme in my life is also found in Scripture: God does impossible things through hearts that are willing to surrender to His possibilities.

> But Jesus looked at them and said to them, "With men this is impossible, but with God all things are possible." (Matthew 19:26)

Just as we talked about the shadow of marriage, and of pregnancy, flowers are shadows here too. The flowers that God has me tend to are not of the hydrangea and daffodil variety, but are the souls growing around me. Just as varied, just as delicate, just as lovely, the women (and some men) around me are grown up from seed, striving against weeds and weather. We live in harsh times. While some souls are heartier than others, we all need these basic elements to thrive: air, sun, water, and soil. Some need more of these than others, and God is not only the Creator of all souls, but the Master Gardener for our growth as well.

That God trusts me at all, ever, with the heart of one of His own continues to be a mystery to me. I remember where I've been, who I've been, and often feel completely disqualified to show up in another person's story. But He is with me, and I am with Him, always. Together, He and I are moving into each day with an eye for the flowers: how to plant seed, how to water, how to nurture, and eventually, how to help them flourish.

A TIME TO CLOSE, A TIME TO OPEN

What I'm about to say will seem untrue, but I mean this with my whole being: I am grateful, now, for infertility. I know, it sounds like something I "should" say in a book like this, but don't really mean. I didn't say it on Day 1. I didn't say it in Year 1. But I am able to say it truthfully today.

When I look at the role of infertility in my story, I see it as a gift that rescued me from a life locked up in small story living. When infertility broke through into our marriage, it stripped me of shadows I could have easily gotten caught up chasing. I could have become more focused on my body, more dependent on it to do what I want it to do. I could have become obsessed with shaping my family into the ideal I carried in my mind, getting the numbers and genders just right. I could have looked at my children as symbols of my own worth, rather than as humans in need of someone to nurture and guide them into God's Kingdom. I could have become consumed with having the latest and greatest children's things, rather than conforming the tiny soul forming within a little frame with the greatest gifts of grace.

I sincerely believe now that had my womb never been closed, my eyes may have never been opened to the vision for motherhood God has for each of us in His Kingdom. There is an epic story unfolding all around us; a Kingdom is being built up in a land far away, and there is a work for us that we are specifically created to complete. God has made us in hidden wombs for a special purpose, and Has given each of us a name. He is preparing His children, even now, for our journey Home.

If not for infertility, I may have never shifted from my humanity to my spirituality, and it is in holding them both that I move into my destiny. Yes, my little dream of bearing children died. I won't have that experience in this body. But, my dream didn't die and fall to the earth ending all hope of family, life, goodness, and meaning. In that death, God resurrected for me a new dream! A new life, with new hope of a new family has come alive to me that will outlast any children I could ever birth on this earth. Where a large table sits in my dining room some nights with empty seats, my farmhouse table in Heaven can brim over with chatter and storytelling. Mouths will be filled that tell of my life touching theirs, our stories weaving together. We will sit and laugh in amazement for how good God has been to us.

Friends, there is a time for each of us to choose to shift from our humanity to our spirituality, and make a decision for how we will spend our days. In her endorsement for Jennie Allen's book *Restless*, Christine Caine said:

> Deep down we know we were made for more than where we are and what we are doing right now. There is something to be birthed through us. Whatever our history has been we know we are somehow a part of destiny and we want to play our part in realizing that.[8]

Infertility was, for me, a wake-up call to remember this is not my Home and I am not my own. I have a purpose in this life and I don't want to miss it. Not anymore. Yes, there is a time to weep, a time to receive counsel and compassion from others as we find our way to hope. But a day will come when it is time to pick up our mat and live our meaningful life. I carry my mat of infertility grief with me now, yet am choosing to live my meaningful life with my eyes opened wide to a motherhood that looks missional, even at times militant, but always dependent on God's grace and love at work in us. I feel rescued from barrenness, thanks to infertility. I feel invited into the greatest calling a woman can receive because I carry Jesus within me. Every day is new with Him, and I can expect Him to bring life through me at any moment.

There is no spiritual menopause in God's economy. If you are with breath, you are with Child.

And for those who are physically past childbearing years, tempted to think this is not for you, let me make this plain: there is no spiritual menopause in God's economy. If you are with breath, you are with Child.

See, without infertility, I may have missed the real thing *motherhood* is because I am daily prone to chase shadows. I may have never realized the bigger dream God has prepared for me! Thankfully, God caught my attention, and maybe now He is catching yours, too. Oh friend, may you realize the bigger dream God has prepared for you. What do you want more than anything? Is it a shadow, or the real thing? Your life will shape around what you want, whether you realize it or not. Shadows can leave any woman feeling barren, while the real thing never disappoints. God is right now offering you the same hope of rescue from a barren life, the same invitation into a life so much fuller than maybe what you have dreamed. A life spent in meaningful ways that will matter not just in this life, but in the life to come too. He is offering grace enough for you to say "yes" to this way of life:

> *Yes, God.* I will let go of my dream (to bear that child, to meet that spouse, to heal in my body, to have that relationship, for that house, for more influence, for that business, etc.). I will let it die in Your sovereign will, trusting You can resurrect a bigger dream based on Your design for me.
>
> *Yes, God.* I release the belief that I have nothing to offer and take up the truth that I have the unstoppable seed of Christ within me. I have the power to bring life from death because of Your power in me.
>
> *Yes, God.* I am letting go of the things others have said about me that do not bear life, and I am going to listen to what You say about me.

If this is you, then you are ready to move on to the last part of this book, with hope. Don't worry if your faith feels small, friend. You will discover that the power is not in the size of your faith, but in what your faith is in that makes the difference.

All it takes is a seed.

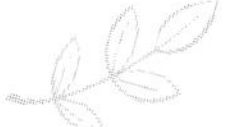

Anna's Story

I never really wanted kids. I didn't dislike them and was actually good with them, it just wasn't part of my dreams. I wanted to be an English professor, live in a big city, and marry a handsome man who shared my love of Shakespeare, football, fine dining, and junk food. None of that happened. I married young, didn't graduate college, and divorced young.

I had strayed from my faith and at twenty-six found myself unmarried and pregnant. My boyfriend and I thought getting married would be best. At my first doctor appointment, a heartbeat couldn't be found. An ultrasound was ordered, and although I was far enough along, still no heartbeat. I went in for a routine appointment and left knowing my child was dead inside me.

We married anyway, but the next several years were filled with heartache. We had no baby, no Jesus, and no real foundation for our marriage. Vows and hearts were broken. And I silently ached for the child I didn't get to know. I kept that and many things to myself, as did my husband. We were strangers who had lost the one thing that brought us together.

Then after years of verbally and emotionally abusing each other, along with the devastating death of my husband's brother, we began searching. We both came back to faith and began making Christ the center of our marriage. For the first time, we were feeling true joy and wanted a family. We tried getting pregnant for a few years, but it didn't happen. In 2013 at my annual appointment with my gynecologist, she recommended I track my ovulation to help determine how to move forward. I did and at my next appointment I was certain she would prescribe an oral estrogen modulator and that I would be pregnant in no time. I gave her my findings and she agreed, "I think Clomid might be the answer." I was elated.

The rest of the appointment went routinely. She made small talk as she conducted the physical. We laughed at a story of her at the grocery store. Then her facial expression changed. During the breast exam, she felt a lump and although she tried to hide it, she knew it wasn't benign. Our plans went from prescribing Clomid to ordering a mammogram, then on to an ultrasound and biopsy. Seventeen days after the appointment, when I thought I would be on the verge of motherhood, I received the news that I had stage II triple hormone-receptor positive, invasive ductal carcinoma. Breast cancer.

The next year and half was grueling. Surgeries, chemotherapy, radiation, and hormone therapy. Countless pills, doctor visits, and sleepless nights. After it was over, my new normal included taking an estrogen blocker—not a modulator—to stop my body from making estrogen and for killing any that may be stored in my bodily tissue. During cancer treatment, menstrual cycles usually cease because the body is dealing with so much already and the reproductive system isn't needed to survive. Or so I'm told. It sure felt like I needed mine to survive. I felt empty with it not working.

Eventually my menstrual cycle returned, and with a vengeance. It lasted nearly the entire month, the cramps were unbearable, and the bleeding was uncontrollable. After several months like this, my oncologist began to worry that if I continued to have these menstrual cycles, then I was definitely creating and storing estrogen—meaning that if there were any cancer cells left in my body, they were most definitely being fed and would only grow from there. I had no choice. If I wanted to have a higher chance of never fighting breast cancer again, I had to have a radical hysterectomy. It was a quick, out-patient, routine surgery. That was it. So at thirty-six years old, I woke up with no ovaries or womb and in full-blown menopause. Although it would've been a long shot before, my dreams of carrying my own child were now most definitely gone.

That was over three years ago now and I wish I could tell you that I knew God's plan for me. We don't feel a nudge to foster or adopt, at least not yet. But I can tell you that God has given me peace, no matter the outcome. And in the meantime, He's allowed me to mentor some amazing young women. And this doesn't just make me happy. It brings me joy. There's a big difference.

UPROOT

What are you holding on to that is holding you back from saying "Yes" to God and possibly a bigger dream that He has in mind for you?

PLANT

Dream a bit about how God could use your suffering as a means of grace, comforting and strengthening others in their suffering.

PART THREE

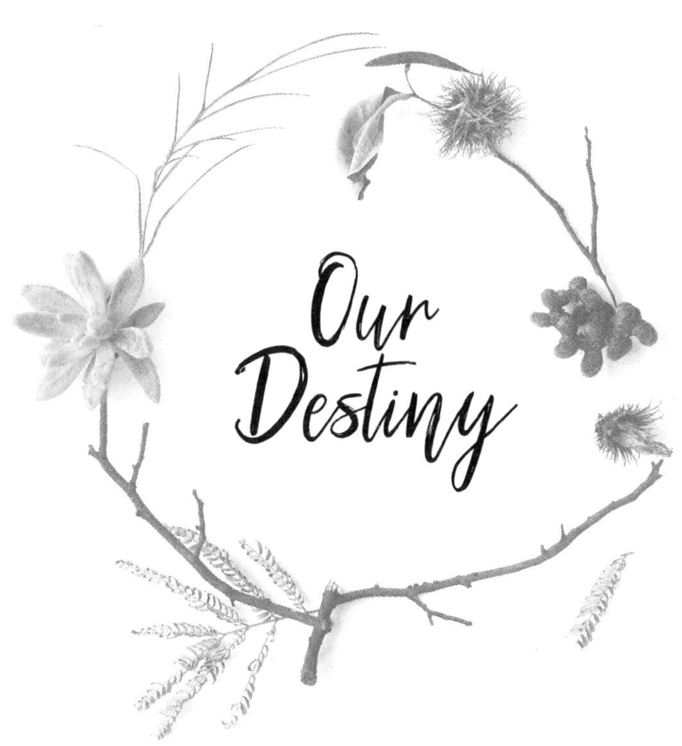

Our Destiny

CHAPTER 10

Plant Small

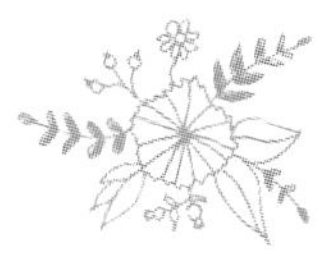

Let us not become weary in doing good, for at the proper time we will reap a harvest if we do not give up.

—GALATIANS 6:9 (NIV)

The looming work of breaking up a wide fallow field before planting season could feel anywhere from overwhelming to thrilling, depending on your personality. I tend to lean toward overwhelming. Like at New Year's, for example. While some are blowing kazoos and clinking glasses of champagne or sparkling cider, I'm tearing up remembering all the events of the last year, imagining all the trials hidden in the new one. The thought of moving wisely through a new year with peace is one I have to set my mind on by faith, or I'll "become weary in doing good" in this life. I can forget that we made it through the prior year one day at a time with Jesus, and reaped a harvest, so we can trust Him to do it with us again.

When I set my focus on the harvest, it makes the slow work of trusting God each day more hopeful. In fact, it is in the mundane daily preparation and simple seedtime season when the work of God in us forms the life we are going to share with others later. The daily work of preparation is necessary if we are going to experience harvest of any kind. And since this preparation and seedtime is where we will spend much of our life, we might as well befriend the process!

THE SEED SHADOW

As you probably know by now, seeds are a type of shadow, too. Picture it this way: a seed is an offspring of a parent or host. When sown in the ground it finishes its work by dying. Out of that death more life can take shape, grow, and break through the darkness into light. In time, there can even be a harvest from that one seed. Paul referred to Jesus as a kind of seed. Jesus was the promised offspring of God, sent to earth by God to live, die, and rise again (Galatians 3:16). While we can see how from His death and resurrection more life is made possible for those who trust in Him for salvation, this is not the kind of seed I am talking about here. There is another "seed" referred to in Scripture that we receive and sow that also comes from God.

The message of Christ, or the gospel, is itself also referred to as a seed. In the parable of the sower, the word of God is likened to a seed (Luke 8:11). As people hear this gospel, the message of Christ, and trust in Him for their salvation, they too can experience eternal life from God. Life from death—harvest from seed. For the purposes of this book, this latter use of the word "seed" is the kind I am referring to: the gospel we receive by hearing and sow by sharing with others. When God gives us eternal life through the gospel, we also become the bearers of this good seed, and can offer it to those around us. We cannot make others believe, just as we cannot make plants grow. This is a mystery, especially to me! God does not call us to bring a harvest of those who believe, because He alone can do this work. What He does call us to do, though, is to *plant small.*

Planting small seeds of faith as we go along in our lives can look different for everyone, but essentially it is the way we share what Jesus has done and is doing in our lives. We tell others what we have witnessed of Jesus and point to Him for our hope. Often we even sow this seed in the hearts of fellow believers, and in our own hearts, so we also continue to grow in our faith! It may be that the seed we sow will yet require others watering it over time, either before someone comes to new life by faith, or a believer grows in spiritual maturity. It may be that we never see the fruit of it. Only God knows the plans He has for our hearts and lives. But the size of the seed we sow doesn't matter. We can plant small with faith in a big God who can multiply one tiny seed into an everlasting harvest.

BREAKING UP THE FALLOW GROUND

As I reconcile myself to my limits in this life, and my dependency on Jesus for life change, I am learning to *plant small* with the seed of God's Word in places where I struggle. I have strived most of my life by trying to change myself, my circumstances, or others through controlling behaviors and radical efforts. If I needed to lose weight, I hit the plan hard. If I needed more wisdom, I'd hit the Word hard. If I needed to be more loving, I'd hit serving hard. I just didn't understand how deeply God loved me, and in my shame and pride, I'd try to fix what seemed "wrong" with me and my world. God has revealed to me over the years, though, that He is in no hurry to "fix me" because Jesus fixed all that was wrong with me by paying my sin debt on the cross.

Out of His wide love for me He desires my freedom from all bondages, so yes, He continually works in me for my change. But even then, He does this little by little in the course of our growing dependence on Him. Just as a harvest is produced over time after preparation and seed planting are all done in the proper season, I too will need to practice patience with myself as God takes me through preparation, seedtime, and some long waits before my heart becomes more like Christ's.

When I use *plant small* in relation to infertility or barrenness of soul, I'm describing *our part* in this transformation from feeling barren to being a world-changing revolutionary. Whether we realize it or not, we *plant small* every day. For example, there is no neutral thought; everything we think has directional value, taking us either toward or away from becoming who God intends us to be. This is why Paul tells the Corinthians to "[bring] every thought into captivity to the obedience of Christ" (2 Corinthians 10:5). Our thoughts flow from our beliefs, and we either choose to believe God or not believe God in each thought we think. This *plant small*, where we personally act to build our thoughts on the truth laid out in Scripture, is revolutionizing. We can actually be transformed into different kinds of people—people who live and love like Jesus by training ourselves to think like Him.

The harvest field is God's Kingdom, which we help grow by scattering the seed of the gospel.

In Romans 12:1,2 we learn that transformation doesn't come from us striving to change ourselves or from controlling all the outcomes through sheer willpower. Rather, it is the work of God in us as we yield our entire lives to Him, renewing our minds with what He says instead of basing our choices only on what we think and feel. Paul exhorts us,

> Present your bodies a living sacrifice, holy, acceptable to God, which is your reasonable service. And do not be conformed to this world, but be transformed by the renewing of your mind. (Romans 12:1,2)

Essentially, we shape-shift from the inside out. As we plant small truths from God's Word in our minds, regularly and over time, we will discover a mysterious metamorphosis within our being. In order to plant seeds of truth in our minds, though, we need to prepare our minds for it. If today you feel like you have nothing to offer, no skill or encouragement, no hope or wisdom, no fellowship or gift, then your mind is fallow ground. Before you can see what God has in store for you, you will need to break up the lies you believe, so you can plant new seeds of truth about who you are and why you are here. Maybe, like me, you need God to help you break up resistance and rebellion in you that is demanding life on your terms.

You may need His help to break up bitterness and unforgiveness over hurts and disappointments in your life. You may need Him to help you break up beliefs that have you locked in habits of destruction, like the believers in Galatia who were lovingly but firmly confronted by Paul (Galatians 5:19–21). You may need help to break up self-pity or loneliness, and make room for the work of Jesus within you, ready to sow seed in and through you! If you are already a believer, God may be moving in your pain this season because He is preparing your fallow ground to take in the seed of His Word in a fresh way that can work a fruitful harvest of maturity and freedom for your soul.

Ultimately, the harvest field is God's Kingdom, which we help grow by scattering the seed of the gospel on the ground of souls around us. In the mysterious will, way, and timing of God, He can bring it to a harvest of believers growing in faith. Jesus Himself likens building the Kingdom of God to sowing seed:

> "This is what the kingdom of God is like. A man scatters seed on the ground. Night and day, whether he sleeps or gets up, the seed sprouts and grows, though he does not know how." (Mark 4:26,27, NIV)

Our part is to sow the seed—the word of God at work in our lives—so others may hear the gospel and believe for salvation, and also for believers who need the nourishment to keep growing. But first, He may be calling us to prepare the soil of our own hearts by breaking up the fallow ground of our flesh so the seed of the gospel flourishes in us. Then we can sow this seed and see God reproduce new life through us.

THE COST OF PLANTING

Though the seed comes from God, and the harvest comes from God, there is a labor in the planting for us. Some call these efforts spiritual disciplines, but really they are small seeds of faith we sow as we grow in our relationship with Jesus. Slowly, in the daily mundane rhythms of ordinary life, we are learning to become new people, like Jesus. Because Jesus is teaching us His ways, we are considered disciples. We are students, apprentices, followers picking up His nuances, His likes and dislikes, His responses to challenging people, and His ways of thinking about everything. This learning involves time listening to Jesus in His Word, living with Him and those in His body, quieting our souls so we can sense His Spirit guiding us and comforting us, and serving others as He prompts us.

Sowing a field is work, so it will likely not feel easy or comfortable at first. At times it will feel like breaking ground, because this is part of the process. Planting takes time and sacrifice. However, when we plant with God, we plant small with the unstoppable seed of the message of Christ! The impossible becomes possible, and even death is surmountable. God can mysteriously take our small sacrifices of faith and bring a return beyond our imaginations. Remember, He can turn even a fallow field into a fertile forest.

THE LEAST LIKELY PLANT TO CHANGE OUR WORLD

As I shared earlier, we went to my brother's house the week after learning that adoption in China was essentially closed for us, and a local adoption of twin boys failed. My youngest niece at the time had just been born, and I was eager to see her, but we had a lot to process ourselves. That first night visiting, both Jonathan and I shared how we were at peace with our family as is and were not sensing an urgency to push forward with another adoption. We both slept better than we had in months, but when I woke up I was hesitant. I wondered if, no *when*, the reality that we may not have more children would usher in grief.

He may be calling us to prepare the soil of our hearts by breaking up the fallow ground of our flesh.

I slowly made my way to the coffee pot where my brother was standing already caffeinated and ready to talk. He gave me a tour, showing me the plants he had bought his wife for her birthday. Half asleep and terrible with botany, I started to glaze over. Then he introduced me to a plant I had never seen before, and spoke words that forever shifted my vision and even changed our lives. There in his entryway my brother introduced me to the plant that could reproduce nonstop, although it was barren:

A mother of thousands.

It was the morning I felt the *least* hope of parenting more children that God gave me a vision for children without number. Not only had He restored in me a hope for family, He showed me where my true hope lies: in the God of hope. My hope is now in the God who resurrects, who is goodness Himself. My hope is now in the God who rescues, who redeems, who displays for His glory those who were destined for destruction, like me! This God, who can turn barren plants into revolutionaries, could take this barren woman and build her into a family for generations.

How does a woman who feels barren grow a family that will live forever? We plant small.

But how? How does *a mother of thousands* fill a yard? How does a woman who feels barren grow a family that will live forever? How do we build when we see so little to work with in our situation?

We *plant small.*

Again, this isn't "small" because we don't have much to offer. It has nothing to do with what we offer or bring from ourselves at all. This whole meaningful journey is simply not about us. Remember, what we plant is not *our* seed; it is the Word of God. It is the seed of His glorious gospel at work in us that we cultivate throughout our lives. And we prepare for it in small ways, over and over, in everyday life. Nothing fancy. No grand gestures needed. Just a heart yielded to Jesus, breaking the fallow ground in our own souls to receive His life, then building relationships with others so we can plant seeds of hope in someone else's desperate heart. We can trust God to bring them to fruition in due season.

Seed in, seed out.

And we change the world.

SMALL TALK ABOUT A BIG GOD

Planting small in the hearts of others doesn't have to be like teaching a theology class. And it doesn't have to look like what *I* do, or what *she* does, or how *they* do it. It could mean sharing stories over coffee, at a monthly get-together, during a lunch break, or while the kids play in a favorite park. Planting small looks like you obeying God with the people in your life. Period. What this looks like is between you and God and could take a million shapes. Remember, God made you uniquely you for a reason. And realize we are not bound by physical age here. An "older woman" spiritually may be in her thirties, engaging with spiritual teenagers or young adults in her neighborhood.

Growing children in God's Kingdom means keeping our eyes and hearts open to nurture hearts that are learning how to live with Jesus. We listen both to God and to the person we are with, trusting that God will deliver the seeds of truth that are needed in that soil as we offer ourselves to Him. Whatever He wants to sow, we can trust He is more than capable to do it.

Discipleship, essentially, is being available to God so He can use us to woo others to Jesus. Discipleship is about listening, watching, and being open for Jesus to transform our lives and our relationships so we all become more mature daughters and sons. Being available for this kind of connection may mean that you need to get up and do something. While I'm not going to tell you what to do specifically, because again this is between you and God, there are countless practical ways to initiate opportunities to *plant small.* I don't know what lights you up, so I don't know how God is going to direct you, but it will involve courage on some level, courage I have needed myself! So let's just accept this and together go into the uncomfortable places for the sake of stepping into our meaningful lives and nurturing the souls around us. Because the question is not whether or not we are mothers, but whether or not we *will* mother. As my dear friend says, "I finally stopped praying to get pregnant and started praying to mother."

Let's be mothers.

BUILDING YOUR FAMILY, SEED BY SEED

In the book of Nehemiah, we read that Nehemiah had a vision for what the temple could become, when he found it in complete ruins. He saw a preferred future that looked very different from the world he was in, and God inspired him to go after it. We need a holy discontent for something in our world today. Something is ruined, a shambles, in need of what we alone have to offer, however small we may estimate that offering. What if we ask God to give us a vision for a future we could enjoy with God, then go after it? We can do mightier works today than Jesus did. Do you believe this? Jesus said so.

> "Very truly I tell you, whoever believes in me will do the works I have been doing, and they will do even greater things than these, because I am going to the Father." (John 14:12)

Jesus said this of His disciples—you and I. But to experience this, we will need to dream bigger. We will need to stop trying to grab shadows, and instead look for the real thing and move toward that, together. It won't be easy; just like for Nehemiah there will be obstacles in the way, and we will have to break up fallow ground in our own souls, but God has a plan in place for us to help build His Kingdom one seed at a time.

I had a Nehemiah moment when I looked at the temple of my soul and found ruin. I cried out on my living room floor to God because I believed barrenness was the real story. The enemy of my soul was planting small seeds of doubt in my mind, suggesting I was missing my best life by not bearing children. Maybe he is doing the same with you, beloved. Do you hear thoughts like these?

You are missing your best life because...
...you don't have a child.
...you don't have a husband.
...you don't have that job.
...you don't have what she has.

Friends, let me speak truth to your souls on this page: get up off the floor. You are not barren. If you are Christ's, you have unstoppable seed within you. Where you and others see barrenness, God sees the potential for revolution.

I am not missing my best life, and neither are you.

I *have* my best life, a life full of meaning and hope where I can *plant small* in countless ways. Harvest is coming, and I'll get to be a part of that celebration. So can you.

I just need help remembering this, especially on days I feel barren.

We all need help remembering we are revolutionaries.

We all need help finding and staying in our meaningful lives, planting small, so we don't grow weary and give up. And we help each other by reminding each other who we are, why we are here, and where we are going.

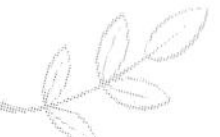

Joanna's Story

Ten years ago, I was in the pit of despair. We had experienced significant loss in our family and the trauma of infertility treatments and miscarriage. It was a dark and lonely time for me and I felt like I had no one to talk to about it. No one seemed to understand my pain. I wish I could go back and tell that girl that there was someone she could be 100 percent honest with who understood her suffering: Jesus! I believe God sent His one and only Son, Jesus, to die a horrific death on a wooden cross for my sins. If knowing you were about to brutally die on a cross, then go through with it, isn't suffering, then I don't know what is.

One of the gifts I've discovered through our struggle with infertility is that I now have deep empathy for others who are experiencing heartbreak like ours. I'm thankful for my retreat from social media during that time, and though I don't wear a T-shirt advertising #infertility now, I do try to make myself available and open to any conversation initiated by a friend or acquaintance. Reaching out to others when I hear of struggle and loss can be difficult, but it almost feels like a natural reflex to me because that simple act of kindness would have meant so much to me back then. I can use the comfort God brought me to comfort others.

While I love it when God uses my pain to help another woman, it isn't always easy to offer this comfort. It is hard to revisit such painful times, but if I can offer another woman a sense of, "Yes, this was very hard, but I survived. God is faithful. He will carry you through this," then the discomfort on my end is worth it. And I encourage others to set healthy boundaries during seasons of struggle. If certain events—baby showers, girls' nights with all the pregnant friends, gender reveal parties—serve as a trigger to spiral down emotionally, then it is healthy and wise to say "no" without an explanation or an apology. You do not have to put on a brave and happy face for all the things, all the time. I wish I had given myself permission to do the same!

Infertility isn't something that defines me, but it has certainly changed the course of my life, strengthened my faith, and shaped me into who I am today. Barren doesn't mean hopeless. You are a masterpiece created by the ultimate Artist. He has a perfect plan for you! Each of us has been given a unique set of circumstances in our lives, and we are not alone in our pain. Others are suffering around us and feel like they have nothing to offer. Our suffering is sometimes not even about us! Sometimes it is the bridge we cross to build God's Kingdom with others. There have been women I could connect with because of my story who I could not have helped without understanding this pain myself.

Instead of focusing on my "barrenness" and lies like, "You're not good enough. You're not good at anything. You have zero to offer others. You're not a *real* mom," I'm choosing to focus on the gifts God *has* given me. He uses me in the midst of my situations, not in spite of them. He uses me through the friendships I form and as I connect women with each other. I practice listening, and take the encouragement I've received to encourage others with the hope of Christ. God always loved me and always will.

Our circumstances are not a reflection of how much God loves us. Just because He didn't let me bear children doesn't mean He doesn't love me dearly and doesn't want to use me in the way I am designed. Or you! Ask God to show you what He wants *you* to do with the gifts and story you have been given... He knows what is best for you.

UPROOT

Are you believing that you have nothing to offer? Do you see yourself as barren, or as a revolutionary with the unstoppable, life-giving seed of the gospel in you?

PLANT

What are some ways God may be nudging you to join Him in breaking up the fallow ground of your soul?

CHAPTER 11

Root Deep

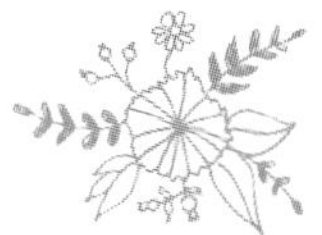

"Blessed is the man who trusts in the LORD, and whose hope is in the LORD. For he shall be like a tree planted by the waters, which spreads out its roots by the river, and will not fear when heat comes; but its leaf will be green, and will not be anxious in the year of drought, nor will cease from yielding fruit."

—JEREMIAH 17:7,8

All plants have a cycle that looks essentially the same: seed, plant, root, and bloom. Once the bloom fades, the growth cycle begins again. No one expects a bloom to come from a seed directly without the planting or rooting—that would be absurd! Always first, a seed is planted. With the seed hidden away in the dark, rich soil, the plant will take root and grow. Over time, with adequate light and moisture and air, only then do we expect a bloom.

It's simple really. No root, no fruit.

To know a plant is to know its roots. When you serve the unique needs of the root system, you can expect blooms in their season. For most plants, roots grow in order to reach water and nutrients to sustain the life of the plant, and can even store nutrients for future use. Roots can grow to varying lengths depending on the plant type. Some roots grow shallow to take nutrients off the top layer of soil where soil conditions are not ideal, while other root systems can grow extensively, like prairie grasslands that grow deep to reach water sources. The deep roots of the grasslands keep grazing animals from easily ripping them from the ground. They are also better protected against wind erosion, and make for easy resprouting after fires.[9] Root systems can grow compact and independent from other plants nearby, or they can grow as one complex root system connected underground, with many shoots rising up, like you see with the stunning and majestic quaking aspens.[10]

The need for a healthy root system is one thing we share with our plant friends.

Roots not only vary in structure and size, they vary in growing seasons. Flower bulbs can take from several weeks to several months to root, though they can be "forced" (or tricked) to begin the growth process during winter months. To have beautiful early spring blooms in the dead of winter, just place a bulb in a dark, chilly environment (like wrapped up in a fridge) for its required rooting season, then introduce it to the warmer temperatures of your home. Voilà—spring comes early for you!

Other root formations, however, are not so quick. For example, on most citrus trees, the first several years of growth produce either no fruit or no fruit you should eat. An orange tree takes about fifteen years to grow to full maturity where it is producing high-quality fruit each year. Not harvesting the fruit for the first few years allows more energy to go into the roots, enabling them to grow deep enough to sustain nutrients. Maturity time for fruit-bearing trees can be shortened, though, through grafting. That same orange tree can mature and bear fruit in only two to three years if it grows from a graft onto rootstock. (A rootstock is a root base from a similar tree.)

To graft, you take a piece of the first-year growth of your orange tree, cut it and expose its flesh, and lay it against the cut and exposed flesh of the rootstock. After wrapping them together tightly, flesh against flesh, you apply a "grafting seal" that works like a glue to help it bond. The grafted branch then becomes a new creation, a new plant. It benefits from the mature root base of the rootstock, and growth comes much faster.

The need for a healthy root system is one thing we share with our plant friends. Where plants have visible fibers that stretch and spread into the soil in search of water, nourishment, and the energy required to flourish, we too have our own fibrous system. In our hunger and thirst for the living water we long for, we stretch and spread ourselves into all varieties of soil. Depending on where we are planted, though, some of us will continue to come up short of the fullness we need to thrive. So from here on out I want to talk about what it looks like for us, the people variety, to root deep in the richest of soil where living water dwells so we can flourish in *our* meaningful lives.

WHO I AM

I just shared about the common practice in agricultural circles that even Jesus cited when explaining how two living vines can become one. Grafting is an everyday technique used by people who tend orchards, vineyards, and the like. I knew very little about it before writing this book, you know, being unskilled in most things scientific and agricultural. Now that I have a better understanding of this common practice, I'm noticing my soul relaxing. Considering that my lifelong quest has been to learn how to relax with Jesus (and not white-knuckle my way though life trying to control all the outcomes), this is no small thing.

As we just learned, when the cut and exposed flesh of the mature vine is wrapped and sealed against the cut and exposed flesh of the immature branch, they become one flesh. Where the branch was once cut off and separate, it is now essentially vine-like through this work of intentional attachment. The branch belongs not because it grew from the vine, but because it has been grafted onto the vine. Adopted, so to speak. The old root system for the branch is gone, and the branch's new nature flows now from the vine.

We can see then why Jesus says of Himself that He is the vine and that we, His followers, are the branches:

> "I am the vine, you are the branches. He who abides in Me, and I in him, bears much fruit; for without Me you can do nothing." (John 15:5)

A branch lying on the ground has little or no root system. It is cut off from its source of life and cannot reach for water, nutrients, or support. What little ability it has to root itself will go unfulfilled in the dry soil away from the vine. Jesus goes on in the next verse to describe the condition of a branch separated from the vine as "withered" (John 15:6). Many today, even believers in Jesus Christ, may describe feeling "withered" because, even though one can be grafted into Christ by faith, it is possible to live as if we are independent of the vine of Christ. We can stretch and spread our thin roots into soils around us that are not the vine of Christ. We can bear shoots of busyness, self-serving, and shadow chasing that drain us of the energy we need to thrive. Simply put, if we are going to grow healthy with God and ultimately bear life, we will need our entire person—body and spirit—grafted (attached) onto Jesus. Jesus puts it this way:

> "If you abide in Me, and My words abide in you, you will ask what you desire, and it shall be done for you. By this My Father is glorified, that you bear much fruit; so you will be My disciples." (John 15:7,8)

If you are unsure whether your branch is grafted onto the vine of Christ, this matter can be settled here and now. The gospel serves to graft us into an eternal security with Christ through faith:

> And you also were included in Christ when you heard the message of truth, the gospel of your salvation. When you believed, you were marked in him with a seal, the promised Holy Spirit, who is a deposit guaranteeing our inheritance until the redemption of those who are God's possession... (Ephesians 1:13,14, NIV)

You have heard the gospel, the message of truth—that Jesus died for your sins, was buried, and rose again. If you believe it by trusting in Christ's sacrifice as sufficient for your sins, then you are sealed by the Holy Spirit, grafted into the body of Christ. In that moment, your branch and the Vine become one. God does that for each of us at the instant of our salvation. We are no longer our own branch striving to produce fruit on our own; we are made new and acquire a new root base in the vine of Christ, mature and lacking nothing. This is Jesus' work, His grafting of us, by our faith in Him.

Our work is to believe by rejecting our old nature through entrusting our lives to Him. As the grafted branches, we died in our flesh by faith, cut and exposed, to be bound to the cut and exposed holy flesh of Christ. We are not the source of life. We do not support the Vine; the Vine supports us.

Branches. This is *who* we are.

But this is something we can easily forget. We can carry on in our relationships and our workplaces, our friendships and our communities, believing we have our old roots, or strive to find sources of life apart from the vine of Christ. We can miss the good news that who we once were is no longer, and who we are now is connected to an unlimited supply of nutrients and life-giving water. We can draw from wells that never run out, like the Samaritan woman recorded in John's Gospel. She needed a way to satisfy her thirst that was complete, healing, and lasting, and He offered her Himself:

I chose to abide in the words of Jesus and in time God flowed His life back into me.

> "Whoever drinks of this water will thirst again, but whoever drinks of the water that I shall give him will never thirst. But the water that I shall give him will become in him a fountain of water springing up into everlasting life." (John 4:13,14)

We will find all we need in our new root system, in Christ. When we miss this, we grow desperate with thirst and run in every direction in search of life. We try to build our own root systems, attaching our identities to things that cannot support growth. With the gospel seed implanted in our souls, and with new growth forming on our grafted hearts, we discover that the only way to grow is to abide in the vine of Jesus.

To *abide* is to "remain stable or fixed in a state."[11] Jesus clarified that as "His words" abide (remain stable or fixed) in us, we can expect to draw from the root source of His life. We don't need to clamor to find sources of life outside of us, or outside of Jesus. We simply need to continue abiding in the words of Jesus, in His presence with us continually, and we will never suffer thirst again.

HOW I SUFFERED THIRST

I know the dry places of trying to root in any place but Jesus. When I was in the deepest seasons of infertility grief, I was tempted constantly to meet my need for relief and fullness of life through the artificial comforts of performance, excess food, and spending. If I stayed busy, or stuffed with high-carb, sugary sweets, or had the cutest new trendy clothes, I enjoyed a temporary numbing from the blinding pain of loss and heartache. I felt abandoned by God, rejected, and cursed, and stumbled over resurrected guilt for sins of my past. The thought of a forever with no children overwhelmed my tender heart, and I often felt withered. It wasn't until I began to root deep in God's Word, as well as in community with others who understood my grief, that I began healing. Just as the aspens root and live in a community, I too needed the companionship of the network of believers who could relate to my journey!

Knowing what we need and receiving what we need are sometimes worlds apart. I didn't feel like receiving God's love from others at first. I wanted to dwell on my hurt and pain, and let my disappointment and anger root deeper until bitterness took hold of me. I resisted Scripture some days out of anger toward God, but by His grace I directed thin prayers to Him asking for a desire to hear from Him. That was my *plant small.* Verse by verse, tear by tear, prayer by prayer, I chose to abide in the words of Jesus and in time God flowed His life back into me. Shoots of new life started to work their way through the darkness of my grief and unbelief into the hope-filled light of day.

As I rooted my mind in the character of God as good, no matter how bad I felt or how bleak my circumstances seemed, I noticed I became steadily transformed by hope. In fact, it was because of the trials that my thirst drove me to root deeper in search of living water, just like the prairie grasslands. The deep emotions I felt were a gift from God in this way. My feelings were and are natural, and I make room for them to show up, but not all things natural are healthy or helpful without boundaries. God's Word was an anchor for me when turbulent emotions were trying to rule my life. I could depend on God's Word to be constant for me, true on Sunday and on Monday.

> "Heaven and earth will pass away, but My words will by no means pass away." (Matthew 24:35)

What I learned about God's character through His Word and my daily dependency on Him was that in addition to His very essence being goodness itself, He was also sovereign, wise, and loving. I held the desires of my heart up to Him with open hands, and learned in Scripture how in control He really is of all the things. He sees what I cannot, knows what I do not understand, and makes sense of what makes no sense to us. When I began to see how He never allowed for anything to happen to His people by chance, but always intended it for some eternal good in their lives and for His glory, I stopped demanding what I thought was best. I accepted He is absolutely sovereign over all creation, which includes me and whatever family He gives me in this life. I even wrote the word "Sovereign" on a stone that sits in my kitchen to be a reminder of God's predictably good and in-control nature.

God's goodness, sovereignty, and wisdom have stabilized me in my grief and in my growing, but the characteristic that is maybe most baffling is His love. God just loves us. With His whole being,

He loves us. At times His love comes through pruning, in trials that do not feel good, but in fact hurt. In this cutting, though, it is always well-intentioned, in full preparation for bearing even more fruit in our lives (John 15:2). God is constantly wooing us to Him, using people, pain, and pleasure, whatever it takes, to get our attention so we will come close and receive the fullness of His love for us. God promises to go before us, to always be with us, to never, ever leave us or forget about us or our pain (Hebrews 13:5), and this includes our dreams and longings. Nothing, not the curse, not our grief and anger, not our heartache and pain, not our pride and sin, nothing can separate us from the love of God in Christ Jesus.

As we learn who God is, we learn who we are, too. Just because we lose things in this life—loved ones, friends, dreams—this does not mean we are losers. In Ephesians chapters 1 through 3, we can learn about who we are in Christ. We now get to practice new thoughts that are based on truth and can expect to find a new life open up to us as we receive the words of God. We root deep as we practice believing:

- We are chosen, not overlooked.
- We are holy and without blame, not cursed.
- We are children of God through adoption, not orphans.
- We are accepted, not rejected.
- We are forgiven, not condemned.
- We have an inheritance; we are not bankrupt.
- We are sealed, not insecure.
- We have the spirit of wisdom and revelation; we are not lost and confused.

- We know the hope of our calling; we are not shooting in the dark.
- We have great power; we are not helpless.
- We are seated with Christ; we are not left out.
- We are alive, not dead.
- We are the saved, not the abandoned, and we have hope forever.

As we root deep in these truths, and grow in the knowledge of God's heart for us, we can find steady ground to stand on with hope that Jesus resurrects what feels dead in us, to new life. Perhaps like the forced bulbs wrapped around in darkness, blooms are just around the corner for those of us in the shade of suffering.

Rooting our identity in God's character is so essential to our understanding of who we are because we will live our lives based on who we think we are. We long for the answer to the meaning of life, and to reach living water. We want to understand who we are, and what we are about. Self-help guides are falling off the shelves for lack of space because we are a people who do not know ourselves. We are learning that we are more than what we do, or cannot do. I am not a barren woman. I am a daughter of God who has an infertility story, as well as a redemption story, and many other stories in my life. In every story, though, I see Jesus pointing me to God's bigger story, where nothing changes who I am.

Even if I could plant the seed of the gospel in my own heart for salvation (which I could not do because I had to hear it from someone else), I cannot root and grow myself apart from the mysterious grace of God at work in me. Just as I had to yield to God's power to save me by faith in Christ, I must learn to yield to God's power to transform me, too. It is incredibly freeing to realize that it is not my responsibility to mature myself. My responsibility is to *plant small* by renewing my mind with seeds of truth from God's Word day by day. The big work of life change ultimately belongs to God. The apostle Paul makes it plain:

> So neither the one who plants nor the one who waters is anything, but only God, who makes things grow. (1 Corinthians 3:7, NIV)

As the grafted ones, we will learn who we are as we learn who God is, since we are now in His vine. No one can teach us who we are better than God. So may we make the decision, if we haven't already, to root deep in the identity of God for our identity, and keep on rooting!

WHY I AM HERE

Why we are here flows from who we are, because God made us the way we are for a reason. Most children are considered "heirs" of whatever small or grand estate their parents may own. When the parents die, the estate passes down to the heirs, or children usually. As God's children, He calls us His "heirs":

> Now if we are children, then we are heirs—heirs of God and co-heirs with Christ, if indeed we share in his sufferings in order that we may also share in his glory. (Romans 8:17, NIV)

As heirs of God and joint heirs with Christ, I have access even now to parts of my eternal inheritance. Every person in God's family receives gifts, like a trust fund, to be used for our good and His pleasure. There are endless possibilities for how these varying gifts can be used to meet needs in our world today. God is infinitely creative, and gives us room to be creative with Him and with the gifts He entrusts to us. I lose the joy of this freedom when I measure my gifts against someone else's. I forget I have freedom, and that my way of using my gifts brings Him great delight. I can forget that I'm not here to be famous, popular, pleasing to people, or live a perfect-looking life. I'm not here to live someone else's life, or even to create a life that pleases me.

I'm here because God wanted me here, and made me on purpose for this generation, for the people I am with, because He is doing something good and wants me to be a part of it. I'm here because I am loved, wanted, and enjoyed by God, free to love and need and enjoy Him too. To use the summary of the Westminster Shorter Catechism, "Man's chief end is to glorify God and enjoy Him forever."[12]

I'm slowly accepting that I'm not here to glorify me, or my family, or my work. God loves me, so I don't even have to actually. What freedom to know why I am here! I'm here to glorify God, to enjoy Him, to use my gifts in the creative ways God has designed just for me so I can bear witness of Him. And hopefully, my witness will cause others to believe, too.

WHERE I AM GOING

In order to build our lives on a secure foundation, our root system must be like that of the grasslands. Our roots need to run deep so we reach the life-giving water we need and will ensure we withstand the inevitable storms, the schemes of God's enemy who seeks to devour us, the strong winds of temptation and philosophy of our generation, as well as forces like fear. If we are expecting goodness, but our hope is rooted in our marriage feeling strong and happy, or having babies, or our children growing up wise and devoted to us; or it is clinging to the people we have in our lives always being with us, or to a dream coming to pass, a business opportunity working out, or us finally getting that house on the coast, then we have shallow roots. Our bodies will feel the stress of our minds not being able to pin down guarantees for where we are going. We will strive harder to control all the variables, but the more we control, the more aware we become of all the variables we lack control over. What does this have to do with living *our* meaningful lives? What does this have to do with our *destiny?*

Everything.

I love the way John Piper states how critical it is to understand the importance of abiding in the vine of Jesus Christ:

> We are not dealing here with something marginal or optional. If we are not united to the vine so that Christ's life is flowing into us, then his words, his love, his joy will be utterly and totally barren. Nothing of any lasting value will come from us.[13]

Did you hear the dreaded word? *Barren.* If we root ourselves in any foundation other than Christ, we can expect barrenness. But if rooted in Christ, we can bear life.

> So then, just as you received Christ Jesus as Lord, continue to live your lives in him, *rooted and built up* in him, strengthened in the faith as you were taught, and overflowing with thankfulness. See to it that no one takes you captive through hollow and deceptive philosophy, which depends on human tradition and the elemental spiritual forces of this world rather than on Christ. (Colossians 2:6–8, NIV)

No matter what your home or family experience is here in this life, it will be perfected in the life coming. Our reality is one of faith for now, because we cannot see it, but in due time we will see it and we will no longer need faith. In this life you may long for children, but you can "overflow with thankfulness" still in the here and now because of the hope that in Heaven you may meet hundreds, if not thousands, of new lives born as a result of your small seeds of faith planted in love! We have no idea just how wonderful Heaven is going to be, and just how impactful our choices today are on our reality there. This is why we are wise to consider our end now, and live *our* meaningful lives with that end in sight!

RESTING IN THE ROOTING

I want to share with you how I got to the place where building God's family became my purpose, even over building my own. If you are in the thick of grief, or feel barren, it could feel impossible to want anything other than the life you expected. I get it. You cannot make yourself love God, or want what He has planned for you.

One of the things people say to couples who are experiencing infertility is to "just relax" when trying to conceive. They add "just" as if it is so easy and natural, the couple *just* forgot to do it. While it may be true that the couple could benefit from a little time away from the constant invasion of options, opinions, and oppressive thoughts that can accompany this journey, diminishing their struggle by suggesting they "chill out" actually can increase pressure to be "okay" with the loss they are experiencing.

If women could only conceive when they had no stress, we'd have no humans on the planet. Stressed-out men and women conceive children every day. I'm not saying stress isn't a contributing factor; it could be. But it is possible to be relaxed and yet still be unable to conceive. I don't know why some conceive and others do not. Call it the grace of God for the stressed, or the will of the Creator of the universe, or the plans He has for us that are higher than ours. What I do know is that apart from God we can do nothing, which includes loving God, relaxing, and conceiving children.

If you have ever felt anxious or frustrated over your lack of spiritual growth or progress in any area of your life like conceiving, perhaps you've done what I tend to do. I "try harder" to follow Jesus in obedience and reach my goal by sheer willpower. The result, though, is that I lose willpower, reach exhaustion instead of my goal, and feel even more pressure to try harder next time. I tell my soul to relax with Jesus, or "abide" with Him using John's language in the verses quoted earlier. But I then carry even more shame for not being more mature spiritually. "What is wrong with me, Lord? Why can't I get over this struggle?" It's akin to asking Him, "What is wrong with me, Lord? Why can't I get pregnant?" I sense silence on the other end some days and wonder if I finally did it—I pushed Him too far to love me anymore. I knew it would happen one day, He'd give up on me. Maybe today is *that* day.

The gospel, though, actually answers these questions for me, for us. The gospel says Jesus died and was buried. He came to do what I could not do for myself. My old identity with its sin and shame was rooted deep in the blood of Christ, all the way to death. Jesus resurrected three days later. Through the gospel, I too sprang up to new life, overcoming sin, shame, and death! I am now a new life grafted to the Vine. This is what I hear now based on the gospel:

> Child, there is nothing wrong with you. Jesus took all that *was* wrong with you to His cross. As for "getting over" that thing, you are already over it. Jesus got over it for you, but you are learning to root deep in the truth of it. Keep abiding in His words, learn to relax with Jesus, and you'll see new growth budding soon. As for "getting pregnant," you are already pregnant, too. Jesus made you pregnant with eternal life that reproduces through you as you share Him with others, but you are learning to root deep in the truth of that, too.

When the gospel soaks deeper into my soul, a mysterious thing happens. I relax. I discover a calm stream flowing on the inside of me that washes over hurts and slights, offering cool refreshing and forgiveness to myself and to others. I feel the fruit of the Spirit—love, joy, peace, patience, kindness, goodness, gentleness, faithfulness, and self-control (Galatians 5:22,23)—forming within me ready to bloom in my relationships. In a sense, then, new life is conceived in the soul that is abiding with Jesus—the one learning to relax with the One who loves us.

Rooting deep is not about fixing ourselves. Rooting deep is ultimately the choice to move toward a person in a relationship. If we measure ourselves in terms of performance in our relationships, we are working, not loving. A relationship is a space we enter with a person, and together sit down to face each other and connect. Our human form is built to face one another, to speak and receive each other with open faces and hearts exposed. Not all relationships will allow for this kind of vulnerability, but our relationship with Jesus is the safest place for us to practice because we are met with unconditional and unrelenting love.

Just as darkness forces bulbs to bloom, trials can bring out rich Christlike character in our lives.

Rooting deep, then, is about learning to abide with the real person of Jesus, to relax in the presence of the Good Shepherd whose main concern is our welfare. Resting in God's love, relaxing in the presence of His Son, returning to the hand-hold of His Holy Spirit, over and over and over, is the work of abiding. Resting is not something many of us are naturally good at doing, though, at least comfortably. I facilitate quiet retreats (you could call them listening retreats since we intentionally set our hearts to tune into the words of Jesus in silence). More often than not I hear from people who confess rebellion and resistance to the abstinence from noise. We are a culture that praises productivity, activity, growth, more information, more input, more fruit, more likes, more, and more. I get it, I'm just as vulnerable to the subtle addiction to noise. But if we keep pushing ourselves for growth, whether it is physically or spiritually, without rooting seasons, without space to practice relaxing with Jesus, we won't experience the fruit our lives were made to bear.

So we embrace rest in the rooting season, for without it we just cannot expect our best fruit.

In the rooting season we quiet our souls long enough to hear God speak to us His words of life. We pause and return to who we are, why we are here, and where we are going. We abide in the vine of Jesus and feel the flow of His words, His love, and His power for us. We root ourselves in the security of our place in God's family, in the companionship of believers. We practice rhythms of life with Jesus like Sabbath, worship, play, rest, work, and more play, so our roots run deep in the joy of God. And in all of this we wait, with anticipation of what He will produce through us, in each season.

THE GIFT OF HARSH WINTERS

I mentioned earlier the hope for those of us who, like forced bulbs, feel the darkness of grief or suffering. Just as darkness forces bulbs to bloom, trials can bring out rich Christlike character in our lives. And the colder the winter, the deeper our souls want to root. Friends, we are living in some cold winter days. All the more may we pull away from the beliefs that lead us to hurry and strive to find security in places other than Christ. Let us turn instead to the warmth and comfort of God through surrender, rooting deep in hope as we stay available to be used for seed planting. May Paul's prayer be ours, for ourselves, for our families, for our neighbors and communities, for the generations coming up under us:

> I keep asking that the God of our Lord Jesus Christ, the glorious Father, may give you the Spirit of wisdom and revelation, so that you may know him better. I pray that the eyes of your heart may be enlightened in order that you may know the hope to which he has called you, the riches of his glorious inheritance in his holy people, and his incomparably great power for us who believe. (Ephesians 1:17–19, NIV)

Just as Job rooted himself in God's character, and trusted Him in his winter months of trial when he could have easily given up, may we too root our minds and hearts in our true hope of redemption:

> "I know that my redeemer lives, and that in the end he will stand on the earth. And after my skin has been destroyed, yet in my flesh I will see God." (Job 19:25, NIV)

Friends, don't go looking any longer for another source of life. It's not out there, it's right here, in the vine of Christ. Root deep, right here. Then, be on watch for the life of God to break through! Keep looking ahead and see like Job how you are coming to a flourishing finish soon.

God will never abandon you. God has planted the seed of the gospel of His Son here in this book, and if you have received it by faith, you are saved. You now bear unstoppable seed and are made to share it with others in your own unique way! God will complete the good work He started in you, but He will not bear fruit without the rooting seasons. This means you will still feel the darkness at times, but take heart and watch for harvest. In fact, may we no longer be ones who are afraid of the dark, because we know Light is always with us.

This is the message which we have heard from Him and declare to you, that God is light and in Him is no darkness at all. (1 John 1:5)

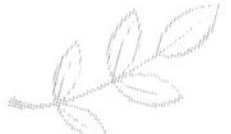

Lydia's Story

After learning I couldn't have kids, I have been brought face to face with my identity issues. My soul leans toward identifying with my job, my family, my health. My failures. The internal struggles this brings with it can tear me up inside, leaving unrest and striving as my norm. But God has gently been bringing me on a journey to re-root myself in Him, and Him alone. When I stop to consider how much God loves me, it recenters my soul. The fact is that He created me *this* way: in this body with these strengths and problems, and with this personality, with its strengths and flaws, talents and weaknesses.

In God's eyes, I am perfect. I am cherished—just like *this*. This perfected me is the joyous result of what Christ did for me.

The loss of natural motherhood is not a hole I need to fill with something else. I can live in this body that will not produce kids, without shame. And my job, while it feels like a calling, has no bearing on my identity either. This is what makes the difference for me between internal distress and internal rest. The difference between self-judgment and self-forgetfulness.

But this is an ongoing journey that God is leading me on, and I fall down as much as I lean into who I am in Christ. Striving pulls me back in easily enough. So I have to continue to center myself on Christ, over and over again. It is this truth of Christ's love and grace that makes all the difference for me. It means joy and trust regardless of my circumstances.

This is who I am, this is what I declare again and again: I am a daughter of the King of everything, completely loved and completely known. This is the truth, and my soul's home.

UPROOT

What do you believe about being quiet and listening to God in His Word, waiting for His Spirit, or fellowshipping with other believers in His body? How are your beliefs hindering you from growing your roots deep with Him?

PLANT

What is one way you can root deep with God this season?

CHAPTER 12

Bear Life

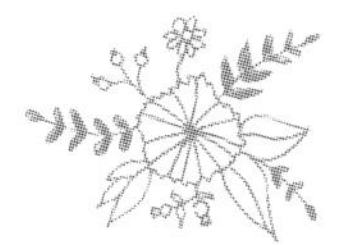

The righteous will flourish like a palm tree, they will grow like a cedar of Lebanon; planted in the house of the LORD, they will flourish in the courts of our God. They will still bear fruit in old age, they will stay fresh and green.

—PSALM 92:12–14 (NIV)

My mother-in-law birthed two sons, and continues to love every moment of being their mom and "NeNe" to their grandchildren. But she longed for a daughter. In fact, she was so positive she was carrying a little girl when she was pregnant with her second son that she painted the nursery bright bubblegum pink. Later, when her son arrived, she loved him dearly, of course. But she had a hard time readjusting her hope.

Many years and several moves later, after her sons were grown, my mother-in-law was excited to finally get *daughters*-in-law. She pursued relationships with us, and has always been kind and generous. Her ability to get around and do things has decreased over the years due to various health limitations, and with both of us daughters working and building lives, I know it wasn't the same as what she had probably hoped for with having daughters. Still, she has continued to pray that God would help her be a good witness of His love and grace to whomever He brought her way. Like when a couple once moved into their neighborhood. Soon after meeting, the wife found a comforting ear in my mother-in-law, and we soon noticed her over regularly to visit. She was wading through infertility grief. Her struggle at the time was just about the only thing she could talk about, and my mother-in-law was about the only woman she could talk to about it. This couple did not know about the love of God, and my mother-in-law was patient to listen, to comfort with words, hugs, and tea, gently pointing the wife toward God.

This *is how we mother.* This *is how we build God's family, through regeneration by faith.*

After a while she began attending church, and then joined Bible studies, amazed at what she was discovering in God's Word. Later, her husband also started in a relationship with God. Today, she is a teaching leader in an internationally known Bible study group and serves with her husband in a local church. She also serves other community organizations and shares the gospel with others any chance she can get through her story, and does so with a contagious joy!

Now ten years later, my mother-in-law is in awe of how God has worked in that situation. Not only did He use my mother-in-law to soothe a woman's heart of infertility grief, but He has drawn both of them into a deeper relationship with Him.

It would have been easy for my mother-in-law to shut down after not getting the "daughter" she dreamed of years earlier. She could have resisted opening her heart to us as her daughters, out of fear of losing her sons. She could have "retired" from sharing God's love with others because her body caused her pain and kept her from "keeping up" with other women in the community. Instead, she chose to root deep in the love of God for her where she was, and planted small seeds of love in the heart of a woman who lived on her road.

My mother-in-law was a mother to her neighbor. That woman even says of my mother-in-law today, "She's my mama." Though that relationship is not biological, biology is not what makes a mother. My mother-in-law made herself available to God: to speak life, nurture, listen, comfort, and guide another woman so she could learn how to have a relationship with God.

This is how we mother.

This is how we build God's family, through regeneration by faith. One soul at a time, one seed of love planted at a time.

She and I were both recently moved to tears recounting God's faithfulness to this woman, but to her own heart too. That God would use us in our limits, in our confined spaces, in our weakness, to bring Him glory and expand His Kingdom is overwhelmingly encouraging. Like I've said before, in God's economy, there is no spiritual barrenness with Christ, no spiritual disability, no spiritual menopause, not even a spiritual death. We are spirit, and the work God does in human hearts is of His Spirit. We simply believe what He says, then do what He shows us to do, and He does the mysterious work of revolution, through regeneration.

My mother-in-law and I were attending a baby shower for a family who had experienced infertility for years. They had decided to foster and even adopt many children during that season. Then by God's providence, she conceived a precious baby girl. We all marveled at the way God had built their family just beautifully, with a pregnancy or not, and we were overjoyed for her to receive another surprise gift! But then her pregnancy became endangered, as the baby was delivered at twenty-one weeks. Sweet "Baby J" had been in the NICU for weeks already by the time of the baby shower, having overcome incredible odds for her fragile little frame. They chose to have the shower to celebrate their daughter's life no matter what happened, and we all had the opportunity to honor God's gifts in whatever tiny packages they come in for us.

We laughed, prayed, ate cupcakes, and watched our friends open gifts. Their kids huddled all around them trying to look over shoulders at what was being unwrapped, wondering what was so special about diapers. Meanwhile, their littlest baby was connected to tubes and wires just miles away in a children's intensive care unit. As I took in the scene, the sounds and the rhythm of laughter mingling with hushed offerings of "we're praying," I witnessed the beauty of motherhood God intended us to enjoy.

Motherhood, in God's design, has little to do with an open womb and everything to do with an open heart. The woman before us *chose* to mother. She didn't wait for her womb to tell her she could; she just walked into it because she had the seed of love ready to share with others, and sowed it with all she had in her. We were the ones blessed to see all the little sprouts growing up around her that day. (Baby J is continuing to grow like the sweetest little flower in the garden, slow but steady, and we pray we get many years with her here, as well as forever!)

IT'S NEVER TOO LATE TO MOTHER

While I wrote this book primarily for women who have experienced infertility in their lives, I have heard from so many women who have felt barren of soul, especially in their later season of life. Even where women have children to lean on and grandchildren to enjoy, I hear the same words coming out of women's mouths who are "past childbearing years":

"I feel like I don't have anything to offer."

"I feel too old, too out of touch with what is trendy."

"No one wants to hear from an old woman."

"Everyone is too busy; no one needs me."

"I don't know the right things to say, or what to talk about, and I have no idea how to tweet or chat or whatever it is *they* are doing these days."

Motherhood, in God's design, has little to do with an open womb and everything to do with an open heart.

I hear from women who believe they are no longer needed. They feel old and dusty, not fresh and vital to the lives of others. All the while, the truth is this group of women holds the most wisdom, the longest history of God's faithfulness, and sometimes the largest quantity of this rare resource: time! Women of older age with a history of following Jesus still carry life-giving seeds of the gospel but are tempted to keep them in their pockets, believing the lie that they are too old to bear life.

At the same time I hear this group believing they are barren, I hear another group of women longing to be listened to, seen, pursued, enjoyed, counseled in wisdom, encouraged in faith, wondering what women who have gone before them have learned.

I hear from women who want to mother, and I hear from women who want mothers.

But who will make the first move?

Several months ago I saw this very dynamic displayed right before my eyes in black and white. I was standing on a stage in another city, sharing a message with a diverse group of women gathered around tables in a church gymnasium. I knew the hostess a little bit, but wasn't sure exactly what the ages would be of women in the room. The event was open to all women in the surrounding area, so usually I prepare for a mix of different generations. This occasion was just that, with girls in their teens and women in their eighties in the audience. By the way, this is one of my favorite scenes. I can see why God delights in the family where parents and children grow together.

The only sad part of this scene, though, was the lack of blending I noticed from the stage. When I scanned the room I noticed several tables in the back clustered with white-haired women, while tables full of dark-haired women crowded at the front. (There were women with other colors of hair scattered about too, of course, but it was striking to me how polarized the tables looked based on age!)

If I had known the community better, or had discussed it with the hostess prior to the talk, I would have shaken them up a bit and made them move around so the age groups could be more evenly distributed for the discussion time. I knew it would make them uncomfortable, and would potentially backfire on the hostess so I resisted, but I felt a sense of loss for what could have been if the white-haired women would have risked showing a little vulnerability to sit with the dark-haired women, or vice versa.

I vowed after that to have this conversation with future event hosts because the possibility for ongoing regeneration in their communities is immeasurable when women wake up to the life of Christ within them. So consider this your official warning, ladies: if you see me coming to your area to speak, be prepared to shake things up and meet a woman you may not have thought to sit by, because she needs you and you need her!

Why? Ultimately, I believe all women have this bridge to cross with each other: we all know shame, and we all need grace. These are the equalizers that can bring any women together, no matter their age, background, socioeconomic position, race, or hair color. But, we will only cross these bridges if we are willing to risk being vulnerable with each other. And women, we are all worth the risk!

EXPECTING JESUS

As women (and men) who want to live *our* meaningful lives and sow the seed of God's Word in the lives of those around us, we will need to consider what we are expecting in ourselves, in God, and in others. You may not be sowing the seed you have because you are expecting rejection, to be misunderstood, to be too old, to be embarrassed, or to not be used by God. This, dear one, is expecting the curse. Satan worked to destroy God's creation, and humanity's resulting sin brought God's curse on the earth. It appeared that Satan had won. But Jesus came to redeem the curse, and give us hope for goodness and growth even in the midst of our weakness. If you have put your trust in Christ for salvation, you have an eternal, imperishable seed of the gospel of Jesus Christ within you that makes you an expectant woman who can enter into relationships expecting... *Jesus.* Instead of being limited by the effects of the curse, we have hope in Christ's finished work on the cross:

> Surely the righteous will never be shaken; they will be remembered forever. They will have no fear of bad news; their hearts are steadfast, trusting in the Lord. (Psalm 112:6,7, NIV)

Of course, we cannot guarantee things will go the way we want them to as we plant small and root deep. The assurance we have of bearing life is not dependent, though, on the response of others. Our hope is in the mysterious hidden work of God in our hearts and in the hearts of others we reach. Bearing life is not up to us, but is up to God. And God can bear life through us even into our old age, friends. As long as we have breath in our lungs, we have the seed of the gospel and God's Word in our soul.

I have wondered, like many do, where I'll be in my final moments. Will my passing be sudden, in a flash through an accident? Or maybe slow and steady, in a facility surrounded only by health professionals, with family either already deceased or busy? I'm not trying to be morbid, but it's something we all think about at some point! I choose to face it head on, though, because another fear that comes with infertility is of aging and dying alone. We see a future with no children and grandchildren to share stories and memories, and to keep companionship with in lonelier days.

I am also never without children and family when I see myself as a mother of thousands.

I used to visit the sister of one of my mom's older friends in an assisted living community years ago, before she passed away. I remember crying every time I left, because I was single and terrified of being alone in my last days with no one to visit me. But in the same way I am never truly alone because of the constant presence of Jesus with me, I am also never without children and family when I see myself as *a mother of thousands*. I have said that I want to make choices relationally today so that I'm invited to as many weddings in my final season as I am to funerals. If I want a relational harvest, now is the time to sow seed:

> Now is your time and now you are here for such a time as this. You will not pass this way again. There is only one now. Eternity is worth the risk. Now is not the time to be demure with the gifts you've been given. Share them lavishly. Now is

> the time to let your life be poured out as ink in an epic story of bold sacrifice and startling courage. —Ann Voskamp[14]

I don't know how or when I will die, but I'm not as afraid of dying alone as I used to be. I'm not saying I wouldn't feel lonely, and it wouldn't hurt. Remember, humanity is a part of our story; our feelings are real and matter. However, our spirituality is also part of our story, and my eternity is real and matters, too. With eyes to see every soul as my potential child, my sibling, my kin by faith, I can have confidence that as long as I have breath I have God's seed to sow that could regenerate new life. I don't want to keep it in my pocket in fear, but sow it with all I have in me, until my last breath.

ONE SEED IS ENOUGH

My daughter recently started talking about how many babies she wants to have some day. We started at 531, but I'm happy to say we are now in the respectable double digits. It has been sweet and hilarious listening to her plans for parenting too. She is going to have her uncle and a family friend "build lots of bunk beds" to house all her babies, which makes sense for space and efficiency. (Her daddy and I are just praying she marries a prince who loves chaos and passionate deep feelers!) While it is highly unlikely she will birth more than twenty babies, most women are born with one to two million eggs.[15] It's remarkable, really. Then with each passing month, the number decreases until that one season when they are all gone. Over a lifetime, she may bring only a handful of little ones to full-term in this world for various reasons.

Again, *every mama has her limits!* And yet, she would never think less of any one of her children just because she didn't have hundreds of thousands more! No! Just as we cherish our one and only daughter under our roof, regardless of what children we *don't* have, she too will cherish each child she raises. Even one child will be worth the hardest labor and delivery to her, just as she has been worth everything to us.

What is true of our bodies is also true for our souls—we all have more potential than we can fully realize in this life, because our humanity will hold us back from fulfilling our destiny perfectly. Our capacity for bearing life with the limitless seed of the gospel of Christ is more than we will fully realize in this life, but what we *do* experience with Him can be worth everything.

As we move along in *our* meaningful lives, we will be tempted to focus on the many children, or many gifts, or many opportunities or blessings others have that we do *not*. This is a trap of the worst kind, and I know it all too well! More is not more, necessarily. Sometimes more is less. Even consider this book you are holding in your hands right this moment. If I had birthed a baby, you would not have these pages before you. If I had birthed a baby, my first book would not have been published. My first book was the fruit of a rooting season in my basement, where I was learning how to weep and laugh again with God. I'm so grateful that story got told, too.

As Maya Angelou said, "The greatest agony is to bear an untold story within you." My redemption story will not go untold now all because I was unable to bear a child. But also, I think about the women and teenagers I've had room for in the space where I wanted more children to fill. I have hugged and shared tears with hundreds of teen girls struggling to understand God's love for them. What a privilege! I could have focused on how I didn't end up birthing children, or adopting more children. I could have confused quantity for quality, and not appreciated the significance of singular blessings. I could have chased the shadow of more and missed the real thing: the one seed that grows God's forever family.

I want you to remember the nature of the unstoppable seed that God has given you. Where some seeds can only be sown one at a time, with a limited harvest, the seed of the gospel can fill a field! Each time it is sown, God can reproduce new life, again and again. His family can grow exponentially, even through one person faithful to sow it.

Now is the time to prepare and to be expectant of life to come, even from us.

Don't bear untold stories, not when they hold the gospel within them.

Tell of the tears, the fear, the disappointments, the heartache, and the God who came in and called you a *mother.*

I'll say it one last time, in case you haven't received this message yet: God has made us mothers, by faith. He has a revolutionary world-changing work to do through us. He is right now bearing life through the unstoppable seed of Christ's love in the hearts of His children. But, and this is a big but, in order to move into this kind of life we must move through and out from our barrenness.

As my daughter reminds me, "Mommy, never give up," I remind you now for your own daughters' sakes: *Never give up!*

> So do not throw away your confidence; it will be richly rewarded. You need to persevere so that when you have done the will of God, you will receive what he has promised. (Hebrews 10:35,36, NIV)

Harvest is coming, soon. Do you not recognize the times? Even now, hope is springing up. This hope is not *of* you, but it is *in* you. Our hope is the life of Christ growing into full maturity in us as He brings the hour to pass when we will be forever united with Him.

Now is the time to prepare and to be expectant of life to come, even from us.

We can today be:

> Women expecting new life…
>
> Women with Child…
>
> Women carrying precious cargo…
>
> Women swelling with hope…
>
> Women watching for goodness…
>
> Women nurturing others…
>
> Women who *plant small*, *root deep*, and grow confident in the hope that we will *bear life!*
>
> We can be women expecting…*Jesus.*

This is not about religion; this is about revolution.

The curse says none of us can bear life. The cross says even the barren woman can be a mother.

Closed womb, meet an open tomb.

Friends, since we are made to be mothers, let us get on with it. There is a time to weep, yes, but there is also a time to sow…and the time is now!

So go, daughter of God by faith, live *your* meaningful life.

Plant small, root deep, and I believe you will become *a mother of thousands.*

Elizabeth's Story

Bear life. Two words that seemed unobtainable after eight years of trying everything to become pregnant. The pills, the shots, the weekly doctor appointments, just to end up with another ultrasound that showed an empty womb. I lost my joy. I lost hope.

Then one Wednesday night our Bible study was on the book of James. During that study I believe Jesus spoke to me, that we were being called to actively take care of orphans. He showed me that I would bear life though adoption and fostering children that were motherless. It took my husband a few weeks to wrap his head around it, but once he did we were a united front waiting on God to show the way. At first, it hurt that we would never know what carrying a baby would be like or see what a biological child of ours would look like. It seemed that during that time of trusting God and following His will, everyone was getting pregnant around me and that stung even more.

Over the next four years we would foster six children. God allowed four of those babies to become permanent members of our family! It was never in my earliest plans to adopt, but allowing God to work through me and heal my hurt helped me see that bearing life just looked different for me. God has trusted me to be the best "mama bear" I can be with Him, to four babies who had no one to mother them. Really, He always intended me to be their mom!

My hope in sharing our story is that you see God has a very special plan for your life. The journey of infertility was one that I never dreamed I would have to go through, but in doing so, I discovered an entirely new world where God needed me. He invited me to mother the motherless. I created life in these babies when all seemed hopeless—for them and for me. I chose joy, and I pray that you will too, wherever God plants you.

UPROOT

Do you still believe you have nothing to offer? No family to identify with, no wisdom or influence, no one needing the hope you have to share? Where is this coming from, and why do you think the enemy would benefit from you believing it?

PLANT

If you have breath in your lungs, God has a plan for your life. If you have trusted Christ with your sins, you are God's child, and He has placed seed in your heart by placing the life of Christ in you. He calls you to share the gospel, which can lead others to eternal life, so in this way we are empowered to continually bear life. There is no spiritual menopause, spiritual disability, or even spiritual death with God.

So what is stirring up even now in your heart to pray? Please, pray it. Write it out. Whatever it takes to give it air to grow. Then, sister, it's time to plant. *You* are a mother, even *a mother of thousands*. You are not the barren woman. *You* are a revolutionary.

Acknowledgments

I have been blessed with many mothers in my life. One being my earthly mother, Barbara, who continues to remind me who I am, why I'm here, and where I'm going. Thank you, Mom, for mothering my soul all these years. My grandmother, Helen, who has already gone to be with our Lord, also mothered my heart. She inspired my middle name and so many brave steps in my life. I miss you, but we will be together again soon. And to my second grandmother, Lilly, who came to love us in her place, we thank God for you. We didn't expect such tender love to come our way after our loss, but God surprised us by bringing you to our family! I hope we have loved you like the children and grandchildren you always wanted to have, because we sure do. I'm so grateful for the ways these women have helped shape me into the mother I am today.

But I am thankful too for the hundreds of women who have shaped my life with their words, their stories, their challenges and comforts, their long talks or short texts filled with truth and courage. There are too many to count, but these are a few who helped this message get into this book…

To my mother-in-law, thank you for modeling for us endurance. You have continued to pray for us, and always seek to serve us no matter how inconvenient it may feel for you. We see your sacrifice and appreciate it more than our lives show you.

To my Aunt Leslie, who has pioneered in our family through some "thorns and briers" but has pointed me to the cross for my hope. Thank you for never giving up, and for leaning into the warm embrace of Jesus.

To the women in my loyal little book club who plodded through the unedited versions of this manuscript in order to serve me with questions, perspective, encouragement, and support, thank you! Allison, Jennifer, Sarah, Amy, Robyn, Jennifer, Angela, and Lauren, you women know how to keep another woman moving forward in her lane. Thank you!

To Lynn Copeland of Genesis Publishing Group and the talented team at Bridge-Logos who thoroughly edited this work and asked me some of the hardest questions, but then presented this story with gusto to the world—you have my deepest appreciation and respect. Thank you!

To the women who put their reputation on the line with their names on this book: Renee, Carolyn, Carol, Julie, Angela, and Lois, thank you for supporting this message and the writer behind it. You have been a sweet blessing to me!

To the brave women who said "yes" to sharing portions of their infertility stories in these pages, I am overwhelmed by your courage and willingness to be used by God to comfort others. You dusted off the old boxes of your memory and heartache to sort out what God could use to help others. I pray you are comforted and strengthened to do this more, to "bear no untold story" and finish your race with joy!

To my community of women with infertility stories who have adopted children, you folded me into the safest huddle for healing, and I thank you. I felt lost in grief and you gave me shelter. I was weary with thirst, and you gave me a cool drink. May God pour out His blessings on your families!

To Mama Joan who reaches across a table to hold my hands in hers, and is quick to share my tears, thank you. You have walked through my married years as a kind and gentle friend, and even though you have great-grandchildren you can see and touch, I know there will be countless waiting for you on the other side of things.

To the woman who bore my daughter in her womb, thank you. I think of you all the time and pray for you often. You are never far from my thoughts, and I pray you receive the love of God washing over you with His comfort and enjoy your meaningful life.

To my daughter, who is already a little spiritual mother, thank you for reminding me how simple the gospel is and how wonderful daydreaming of Heaven can be for us. In your childlike ways, you are shaping your mama's soul. Never doubt your impact, my darling. You have an unstoppable quality living within you, and I will always be cheering you on!

Though he is not a "mother," my husband, Jonathan, has been at times like a father to my heart. Sweetheart, I see God's unstoppable seed in you, too. You are like Abraham, a "father of nations," and this too is all by faith. Thank you for not letting me quit this book. Thank you for pushing me with love, believing in this message. Thank you for caring for women who have felt barren like I did, and for praying they feel the freedom we have tasted with Jesus. Ultimately, we are mothers because we all have a Father who loves us. So too this book for mothers is here because of the fatherly love you modeled for me. Thank you, Babe.

To the One who made me a mother, first by faith in His Son, Jesus, and then through adoption, thank You. You invited me into Your epic story, to grow Your family in quality and quantity, and I'll never get over this privilege. You rescued me from the shadows, from small stories, and from a wasted life. I pray now others look to You and find the love and peace You've shown me.

Take all the glory, Lord . . . it all belongs to You.

Notes

1. "Revolutionary," Merriam-Webster, Merriam-Webster.com.
2. "Revolutionary," *The Oxford Pocket Dictionary of Current English*, Encyclopedia.com.
3. Twitter @timothykellernyc, January 20, 2014, 8:53 a.m.
4. See *StrengthsFinder 2.0* by Tom Rath (New York: Gallup Press, 2007). The assessment is available online using a code found in the back of the book.
5. Judith Orloff, MD, "The Health Benefits of Tears," *Psychology Today*, July 27, 1010 <tinyurl.com/y5u3p5xt>.
6. Golda Meir in an interview with Italian journalist, Oriana Fallaci, published in *Ms.* magazine (April 1973).
7. "Sarah; Sarai," International Standard Bible Encyclopedia <tinyurl.com/y35ze9hf>.
8. Christine Caine, endorsement of Jennie Allen, *Restless: Because You Were Made for More* (Nashville: W Publishing, 2013). I highly recommend this book as a primer for discerning what "more" God has made you for uniquely.
9. "Plant Adaptations," Biology of Plants <mbgnet.net/bioplants/grass.html>.
10. Hannah Ettema, "Tree Profile: Aspen—So Much More Than a Tree," National Forest Foundation, March 21, 2014 <tinyurl.com/jcagdlq>.
11. "Abide," Merriam-Webster, Merriam-Webster.com.
12. "Westminster Shorter Catechism," Center for Reformed Theology and Apologetics <tinyurl.com/y6t5l794>.
13. John Piper, "What Does It Mean to 'Abide in Christ'?" Desiring God, September 22, 2017 <tinyurl.com/y3dlct3x>.
14. Ann Voskamp, endorsement of Jennie Allen, *Restless: Because You Were Made for More* (Nashville: W Publishing, 2013).
15. "How many eggs does a woman have?" WebMD <tinyurl.com/y54nncsz>.

STILL NOT CONFIDENT IN SHARING YOUR REDEMPTION STORY WITH OTHERS?

Order Heather's book
All the Wild Pearls:
A Guide for Passing Down Redemptive Stories
and experience writing your own story as you see hers unfold!

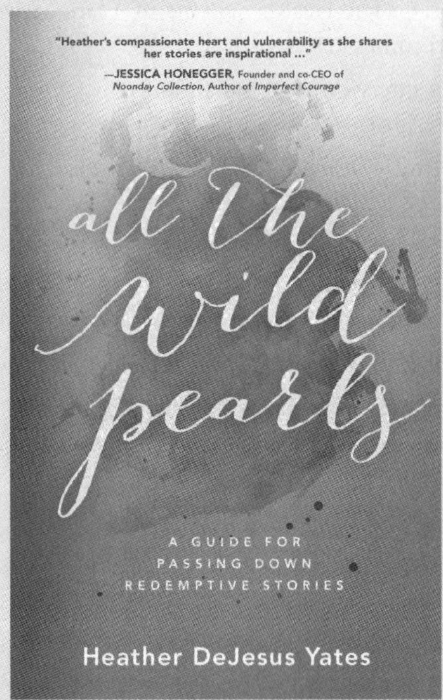

You can find all of Heather's books and other resources at
heatherdejesusyates.com
or you can purchase her books at CBD.com and on Amazon.